"Sifu Slim's narrative is a fresh approach to body-mind fitness and is so full of common sense, logic, and promise that following his philosophy and program could very well change your life."

—Wendy Allen, PhD, clinical therapist,
co-author of "The Business and Practice of Coaching"

"Though people talk about the Paleolithic diet and the hunter-gatherer lifestyle it is rarely presented in context. This book reveals extensive anthropological and historical evidence that provides that context and enlightens the reader of the significance of being true to our own cultural and biological heritage."

—Dr. Tom Rook, chiropractor for more than 30 years

"Sifu Slim's book couldn't be more timely for the direction we as a society and planet are heading in community and health. Whether you are new to the movement of living 'natural' or someone who has long been a health advocate, Sedentary Nation fuels a spark to reshape yourself and the world around you."

—Isaac Osborne, ASI, AET, posture alignment therapist,
owner of Motion Unlimited

"This book hits a home run in capturing the problem of our era. More than 20 years ago, before I went into practice, I thought most of my patients would be people who did physical labor. The opposite is the case: Desk workers have more problems because they don't move all day. The irony is the more educated move less!"

—Dr. Donald Liebell, D.C., B.C.A.O., Va. Beach

SEDENTARY
NATION

SEDENTARY

The
Answers
Are Found
In 1910

NATION

*SifuSlim's
guide to getting off the sofa

Paperback ISBN: 978-0-615-39070-3
eBook ISBN: 978-0-9911829-1-6

Printed in the United States of America

Cover Design: slyfoxstudio.com

More by Sifu Slim

The Aging Athlete—Elite Athletes Reveal Their Secrets for Life

For our ancestors, whose lives can teach us adaptability,
determination, and doing the right thing.

I'd like to express my gratitude to those who have
historically preceded us and to those who have read and
commented on this book for their knowledge and experience in
adding to our better understanding of the serious problem
of wellbeing we're facing today.

Liability Waiver

The lifestyle advanced in the following pages has worked for me and a number of people I have been privileged to learn from or mentor. It is both a compromise and an adaptation. These days, most people in the West spend most of their lives taking up static space—standing or sitting—not moving gracefully or vigorously in an anatomically friendly way. It's simply the sign of the times. Some of us have chosen not to sign on to those times.

The compromise one can choose seeks to relieve the body of much of its sedentary reactions—most notably pain and dysfunction—and the mind of its stresses and pressures. Visits to the psychological counselor are way up as is the use of psychotropic drugs. My findings, which psychological counselors acknowledge, suggest that sleep disorders are driving lots of this. And, what do you think might be driving poor sleep?

One leading premise is that poor physicality, poor diet, and excessive material world madness leaves us wired at the end of the day rather than tired. Asian health practices and Ayurvedic principles can both be applied to this staggering situation.

The countermeasures found in this book are based on diligent interaction with wellness experts, the honing of a personal wellness practice, wide reading, and years of contemplation. Should you have any reservations about being able to travel through the pages and coming to some sensible decisions that might benefit your own particular wellness, please put this book down now.

This is a book on living more naturally in our busy, modern world. It takes up sedentism, self-mastery, fitness, and the wellness mindset. This book does not advocate rapid transformation or excessive heavy-duty effort. You should not go out and attempt to get fit and well in a week or a period that is too short for the reality of your current health condition and schedule. That said, if your health is currently compromised, you shouldn't wait until you are diagnosed with arthritis, nerve damage, gallstones, or type 2 diabetes before you make some changes. Waivers that say to check with your physician before undertaking any wellness changes are helpful and I suggest the same. Make sure your physician does a comprehensive evaluation and knows your complete history.

Attend to that before making any dramatic changes in your activity level. If you aspire to get off the couch and begin a walking program by walking your child or grandchild to school, the best person to consult with before venturing out onto the road is the crossing guard.

Contents

Summary

Sedentary Nation recalls pivotal moments of the history of physical movement. Despite modernism and the decreasing use of the physical body, this book shows how almost anyone can easily benefit from a program that has a payoff of improved health, youthful look and energy, better sleep, and clearer thinking without the physical toll and battle fatigue that often accompany other approaches to wellbeing and fitness.

Expanding on that, the author details how, as Chinese philosophy explains, you can change your thinking and the body will follow. By sharing knowledge and practices from those he respects the most and cites throughout the book, including Jack LaLanne and Bruce Lee, Sifu Slim describes his own journey of self-mastery. Sedentary Nation is the result of several hundred interviews and over a decade of research. It stands as both wellness guide for the busy, modern era and humorous memoir of a life spent living the wellness walk.

What do electronic gadgets have to do with sedentary lifestyles? Answer: Everything.

You may be thinking that prostrate means lying face down. It does. It also denotes "completely overcome and lacking vitality, will, or power to rise."[1] People complain they are so wired and tired these days. Some of the sluggish don't even want to get up to go to the bathroom. Loads of people do admit they'll make the effort to move in the direction of the freezer and microwave. Exhaustion breeds sedentism and sedentism itself breeds further sedentism. Sedentism also lends itself to excessive eating and drinking. We are programmed, and in fact we're adept, in consuming food and beverages, especially the easy-chew food. Food marketers, food scientists, and our own intensifying addictions easily arouse the impulse-reward centers of the brain. The pursuit of food, and other necessities like firewood, water, and shelter, is what kept us doing physical movement for eons. Now, because of sedentary jobs and other "conveniences," we are no longer mandated to move.

The majority of Westerners can spend more than eight hours per day on digital electronic gadgets, both for work and play. What is the number of hours you log?

The answers to many of the problems of inactivity, diet, lethargy, stress, and relationships are not easily found in the millennium. Yet they're readily observable in 1910, a time of movement in relationship to food, family, and work.

The move to wellness is a journey, not a destination. This book invites you along for that journey.

Definitions with Comments

muckrake: to entertainingly and provocatively expose the ills, evils, and reckless behavior of individuals and entities in the hopes of reform. (Besides sedentary lifestyles, what else troubles a muckraker these days? Being stuck inside drywall for far too long and the general dumbing down of society.)

discernment: the wisdom it takes to be able to part the clouds and see what's beyond.

irreverence: a satiric lack of respect for what is considered proper, appreciated by many with good discernment and a love of artful muckraking.

fit: a person with an optimally functioning body and mind and who maintains both with a daily practice and irreverent indifference to anything that seemingly prohibits fitness, like a packed schedule in an over-programmed world or bars on a prison cell … which can be synonymous.

well: a fit person who takes care of themselves and doesn't suffer from disease. Those people who suffer from disease can still practice pursuits of fitness and wellness. (This word is the principal reason I started on a life of pursuing health in all that I do. Known as a semi-sickly child, I was not willing to settle for a life of sniffling and biomechanical breakdown. I made vitality and health my life's work.)

deep pockets: a good thing to have before you buck the system by writing muckraking nonfiction.

excuses: (about fitness avoidance or anything else that detracts from training or doing the right thing): The Marine drill sergeant might harshly bark, "Excuses … save 'em for the undertaker."

a good coach: something we all need. When you have finished with this book, a number of you may decide to sign up for ongoing coaching with the right person for you. (We all benefit from this; even good coaches need coaches. I have known some coaches who are so busy they don't take time out for their own health, healing, downtime, and family time. Some have passed away far too early in life.)

Is your current lifestyle working for you?

Is what you are doing getting you what you want?

Wellness is not a checkup, a shot, a new diet,
or some pills. Wellness is a lifestyle.

When you want to take up wellness, where should you get your wellness information?

This is the biggest challenge an interested reader, author, journalist, or blogger confronts. There is so much information out there, much of it erroneous or biased. The volume of health information is said to double every four years. If you click on a topic, it's easy to land on a page that is offering a product or subscription.

My advice:

1. Read books and articles from sources not beholden to conglomerates. Nearly every large study is sponsored. Find out who's paying the bills and why. Remember this adage: *the media has never met a new study it didn't like.*

2. Find good websites that aren't simply hyping products.

3. Attend lectures by knowledgeable professionals in the field.

4. Watch documentaries that enhance your intellect and touch your soul.

5. Develop your own intuition; it will be your best guide.

Why Should You Listen to Me?

First of all, I care. Second, what I do works.

Mainstream I'm not; and I like to see that as a positive. As far as lifetimes go on Earth, my immediate one started with a lot of resistance to the status quo.

The world was unwell to me; that perception was overwhelming. At a very early age, this culminated in an undying interest and commitment to wellness. We Westerners were simply and blindly accepting too much of a new culture of excess. The current generations were falling prey to excess consumption encouraged by invasive marketing and unprecedented increases in standards of living. Appearing on the scene were human beings turned into walking billboards. *Should mass-manufactured beer and soda logos grace the faces of our favorite T-shirts? Should our playgrounds be sponsored by soda companies? Should our exercise regimes be held indoors?* This made no sense. We had been duped; people had rolled over and given in to the power of money. Why do you think fake powdered juice drinks started replacing lemon aid at refreshment hour around the mid 20th century?

Then there's our infatuation with information, entertainment, and the lives of others. *Should we have TVs going during so many of our non-working hours? Should we know more about the lives of the stars than we know about the natural world, history, and the history of ancestors of our own family?*

We seek out empowerment and therapy because life is full of events that are both unpleasant and absurd. Setting out for achievement, yet beset with addictions and inadequacies, we may be given a list of steps. Until we master those steps, goes the logic, we can't thrive or even keep from going bonkers. Significant numbers of people say they're not happy. The numbers vary on this but they're generally over 15 percent in the West. The numbers of people experiencing significant stress are much higher.

The experiences of primary and secondary school teachers illustrate just how difficult it is to deal with people—other adult staffers as well as the young people. Then there's the increasing workload generated by the modern age's culture of liability and reporting. Some 40 or 50 percent of teachers are said to leave the field within the first five years. Why is this particular career so difficult? Personalities, hormones, and energy levels vacillate and it's often a tightrope walk to make it to the end of the day. Often unassisted by other adults in the classroom, a trained teacher receives a new crop of young people each year. Significant numbers of these students are increasingly unfit, digitally addicted, and suffer poor nutrition. On a continued basis, teachers are required to learn additional protocols to follow. Of course teachers are not the only part of the workforce showing displeasure, anxiety, and blown fuses. Most workers have their gripes. Added up, the gripes may lead to a tipping point which causes many of us to leave our jobs, enroll in counseling, or simply suffer with various degrees of unease.

New books and research studies take up the subject of happiness. The brain chemistry is quite remarkable. With high-tech brain scans, neuroscientists can see moving color images to plot how our brain chemistry is being driven—mostly by the unconscious mind. Eighty or 90 percent of what we do, according to some experts, is controlled by the unconscious mind. Some suggest that evolution has simply programmed us that way. On the surface, that seems to throw a lot of rational mindedness out the door. If the unconscious is running the show, how can we make rational decisions?

The Sniff Test

If, as the saying goes, we are often our own worst enemy, does this mean the impulses that are driven by our subconscious are irrational? Is it irrational for a woman to want to select the correct man by smell or by some inner acuity in her subconscious? Throughout known evolutionary history, the woman has born the children and been the principal caretaker. If she chooses unwisely or unluckily, the man could become absent and she could be stuck with either going it alone or having to choose a new mate in a time of crisis. Or, the original male mate could remain at the location fostering additional friction.

Some health professionals hold that ninety percent of illness is driven by the unconscious mind. Is your unconscious mind creating havoc? Are we helpless sufferers of our biochemistry, worries, karma, and spirit? In a paradigm of potential helplessness, do some need substance counselors, shamans, spiritual guides, and psychological therapists to be at their side at all times?

If that sounds like overkill to you, how about some simplicity in the form of rational willpower? If you're fine with that offer, here's the battle cry: Do the right thing despite your addictions and long-term patterns. Do the right things despite your psychology. Is your conscious mind being overpowered by your unconscious mind to the point it's creating havoc. If so, fight back, reprogram it, then let it go and move on. Here are some straight answers sent straight from your strong-willed ancestors. If you don't like to walk, walk anyway. If you don't like to run, run anyway. If you don't like to eat right, eat right anyway. When you get well, you will be gliding through parts of life, not stumbling.

I've stumbled plenty. Once upon a time, despite an obnoxious TV addiction during early adolescence, I got off TV cold turkey. At another point, in my early 20s, despite a college degree and some enthralling life experiences, I realized how uninformed I was. A sixth sense and some vacant space in my cranial acreage was urging me to acquire more knowledge and experience. (Wisdom is an entirely different subject.) So, I began to inform myself and sign up for new activities. During these initial years of self-study, I attended a think tank held at a convalescent center in Sacramento, California where I had moved from Paris, France—a town steeped in philosophical fitness. There I sat, in these deep conversations, comfortably ill at ease knowing I was easily the low person on the group's intellectual pecking pole. Embarrassment to be able to contribute so little pushed me to at least develop some attentive questions. The informed others could speak at length about history, politics, big business, and cultural trends. It was as though they had spent half their lives in the closed stacks of a university library and the other half in café debates with a group of Parisian scholars.

I wanted in. I wanted a higher level of knowledge. A course of reading, watching, listening, dialoguing, writing, and thinking has been an intentional daily pursuit for decades. Since it's an ingrained personal passion, I don't see the course for intellectual stimulation derailing any time soon.

This awareness acquisition program seemed to lift me up and allow me free travel fare in the archives of the imagination. As for wellness, I roll with the active and natural-based approach to lifestyle which has continued to gain ground on the synthetic version. People want sustainable wellness at low cost with no side effects. They want things to work for them. They also want invigoration and fun things that can fill their free time.

Along this wellness journey, others took me aside and helped me realize some of my personal traits. To them, I had a relentless, maverick view. Some commandment, some singular drive and determination, regularly had me digging in and digging deep when things were beyond my initial capacity. Born into the physical limitation of being scrawny and growing up with a bone structure that was and still is slightly out of alignment, I have always had to do daily work just to keep things from breaking down. The physics of a tall, unbalanced posture stuck in a desk and a car, and my early years playing one-sided sports like golf and tennis, is not good. To thrive and be pain free required being attentive to my physical side on a full time basis. Good fortune enabled an early life of healthful meals and I have never swerved off course. There are a few bonuses to being scrawny. The dumbbells I carry around in my car are not huge. Another is it's easier on the trails I hike.

Far from perfect, but becoming adept in the care of the brain and the body, I have handled most of my days with a call to wellness. I have never liked feeling groggy in the morning. Drinking in excess or until late promotes that, so those nights for me are extremely rare. The local traffic police likely appreciate that. The spiritual connection, I have found, also seems to be in part based on not just being, but doing. There is some talk that goes "we humans are created to be human beings, not human doings." I think we're both. Being in good spirits and in a good spiritual place seems to be most obvious when pursuing honorable thoughts and beneficial goals. The better efforts in this regard have helped keep me alive and sleeping well.

Would you like the ability to replace things that drag you down with things that lift you up? Specifically, you can learn to say no to negative practices and yes to the positive. This can become the driving force in your life, and I can teach how to tap into that. The power is inside you to drive by the convenience store and keep on going, despite any urges to flip a U-y to purchase a former favorite treat. This treat is likely what a health practitioner would call a piece of junk. Though junk is junk, I'm not opposed to expressions of rebellion and wildness or washing down a meal or a group meeting with a treat. Do you want treats that are not only tasty, but good for you too? You don't have to be an athlete or even athletic to enjoy an invigorating hike that ends at the store that makes homemade, organic peach pie with a scoop of homemade whipped cream.

As I say this, my taste buds are firing and my right hand is stealthily sliding the top off the dark chocolate-covered raisins from Trader Joe's. You know that dark chocolate is more healthful than milk chocolate, *n'est-ce pas?* It is made of cocoa butter, not milk, and contains more saturated fats, which makes it more filling and less insulin producing. Milk chocolate contains more carbs, including sucrose, which is half glucose and half fructose, thus making it more insulin and fat producing. The other benefits of properly produced dark chocolate made from the cacao bean can fill pages.

What about the bizarre low-fat diet fad of the past five decades? Heck, I never got hoodwinked—by the big powers including the government—into following it. I can only guess these health saboteurs thought we were dumb enough to believe that all of our ancient ancestors were idiots because they didn't have access to low- or no-fat chips, soda, and milk? Think about it, isn't that nuts? I understand fermentation and drinking wine and spirits, but I don't get the idea of drinking chemicals and corn syrup, or milk with the fat reduced or removed? Do you know how many long-lasting calories it takes to work all day in the field or walk 18 miles in pursuit of a herd of elk? You don't get those calories and energy from a bag of denatured corn chips. (One part of the definition being denatured in this case is to change the organic structure of a food so it has less or no nutritive benefits, possibly changing some of the molecules into harmful substances.)

How silly is that to remove the best parts from food? By design, our bodies require good fats, not excessive junk carbs we turn into excess body fat. Our brain also requires a steady supply of fat calories. Historically, our hunter-gather ancestors were fat adapted. Their stored body fat could easily be converted to sugar to fuel brain function and other energy needs. That's how our systems work. Unlike other members of the animal kingdom, we did not adapt to make our own vitamin C. But similarly to other animals, we excel at making our own sugar from fat.

When they introduced their products in the 1970s and '80s, the top low-fat food producers fully realized this mindless diet would create a health meltdown as well as a remarkable profit center. Some of today's food directors and scientists have openly admitted they don't eat their company's denatured food. Now that the low-fat myth has been thoroughly exposed, why are these low-fat products still being offered? Because they still sell. Dietary and weight-loss products, and pharmaceutical repair products—that mostly claim to relieve symptoms—attempt to counteract the health calamities in part instigated by wrongful diets.

The less fat you have in a product, the more quantities people will need to consume to feel satiated. Fat, protein, and nutrient-dense foods curb our hunger. Corn syrup and simple carbs make us want more. Chemicals amp us up and clog us up. The producers are betting you can't eat just one portion of non-fat yogurt. Have you noticed that it's not easy to find whole fat yogurt unless you go to a health food store? Swedish researchers and others have done studies that show whole fat dairy promotes less obesity than low fat and nonfat dairy.

We need to look beyond the labels, and not just accept the latest—and sometimes long lasting—marketing hype.

Have you already figured out what natural wellness is all about? Are you sedentary more than you'd like to be? Do you lack in exposure to the outdoors and nature? In my offer to help with a workable wellness plan, understand that I'm not coming from some elevated place, above the rest. I look out laterally, standing shoulder to shoulder with you—walking together, without pressure. Some people read lots of information, then think a lot, discuss a lot, and test things. These same people sometimes write books which hopefully provides you with an easier access to good information and perhaps new additions to your personal philosophy. The offerings here are an invitation and it'll be up to you to decide if it can fit in your lifestyle. As a coach, my job is easy if I can slow you down for just a moment. Okay a week. Would you give me and some good intentions that one simple thing—one week? One week to go through what I have distilled down to share.

In that time span, you will learn the formula to increase your health and improve your sleep no matter how busy your schedule and no matter how busy your mind. What if our awakened hours are spent sitting or lying down? Daily periods of physical movement counteract lots of the sedentary woes, but, as the latest research suggests, not all of them. You may have heard the claim sitting is the new smoking. Well, it's true and it's not new news. We just waited until recent decades to classify cubicle-itis as a societal menace—and cause for workers' compensation claims. With that in mind, can a full-time, stay-at-home couch potato sue the cable company? Studies done in the mid-twentieth century found that there were significantly higher rates of heart ailments for seated bus and train drivers as compared to the walking and standing conductors.

Physiologically speaking, long periods of sitting cause damage that even once per day exercise appears incapable of surmounting. Simply standing at a high desk—with good posture of course— keeps your body at an improved level of biological activity. Being awake and sitting or lying around, which numbers of people do upwards of 14 hours per day, means we're puttering on ultra low rather than enjoying a healthful circulation. While inactively sitting or lying, our body inadequately metabolizes the glucose we have taken in at meal time. If we snack and consume sugary drinks, this might equate to eight to 12 doses per day.

A remedy, according to some recent research, is to get up and move for ten minutes or at least stand for ten minutes for every hour of sitting or reclining. This isn't perfection, it's a concession we make for a sedentary daily life.

This doesn't mean to avoid a more rigorous schedule of daily physical movement as in a daily workout, walking steps, or some physical recreation. A number of benefits continue long after exercise hour. These include improved muscle and circulatory metabolism; the strengthening of all tissues, bones, and organs; postural alignment; decreased visceral fat (midsection fat); decreased inflammation; cell repair; the release of energy and toxins; and improved sleep, figure, self-esteem, and love life.

My goal has always been to seek out the perfect workout for an able person. It took me until my late 40s to get it. Here's a preamble. If your exercise/recreation plan (or yoga practice if that's the only purposeful physical program you do) is devoid of any these characteristics, anthropologically speaking, it may be lacking. To be true to our anatomical and biological needs, on certain days per week, you would be doing some of these moves. And thus by the end of the week, each point listed would be accomplished.

1. Some weight-bearing portions which means you are standing on the ground. And some hanging portions where you get extension from holding your weight aloft as in chin-ups or bar hanging.

2. Some huffing and puffing: both through high intensity (like sprinting, short bursts, or walking fast up a hill), and level intensity, which is steady breathing like endurance training.

3. Rebounding which means going up and down, weighting and unweighting from your feet. Think bounding or bouncing. Running, dancing, skipping rope, basketball, trampolines, and tennis obviously provide this.

4. A recreational component. Your program can be entirely recreational like badminton.

5. Outdoor exposure to nature and the sun.

6. Generates function, not dysfunction.

At this point I'm getting off my laptop to go out and skip rope for a few minutes.

Wow, that was terrific! I'm back, feeling better, and still feel the blood pumping through my legs.

The old adage goes, *the best workout is the one you'll do*. That's not a bad start. If it's missing above points four through six, it's highly unlikely you'll do it for life. If it's missing point three, your lymphatic system may be working less than optimally. Part of the reason we experience so much sickness in our sedentary society is due to our stockpile of cellular sewage that's not being properly treated. Point two is how we dump our own HGH, human growth hormone, into the blood stream. This is called the fountain of youth so you don't want to miss that one. And without point one, you can suffer weak and degenerative bones. Swimmers and cyclists are trained to do weight-bearing exercises to counteract this. While in zero gravity, astronauts have suffered atrophy and other ailments due to the inability to engage in weight-bearing activities.

The payoff of an active and functional lifestyle is wellness. The wellness message for the sedentary world is to create balance in your life. There is an easy part in all of this and it's definitely on my side of the equation. The easy part for me as facilitator-coach is as simple as unlocking what's already inside of you—your innate sense of wanting to be healthy and well.

Foreword
"A Psychiatrist's Prescription for Getting *Off* The Couch"

There's extensive, mounting evidence that supports what many people have intuitively known ... that we are sitting too much and not spending enough time outdoors for recreation and physical activity. The paths and fields we played on as children are inviting us, so why won't we reach out to take advantage of what nature offers us again?

We humans need to get moving, preferably outside, for optimal health. Our workouts done outdoors may provide more mental, emotional and physical benefits than those we do indoors. Even the color green, which is abundantly found in nature, may improve both mood and self-esteem.

Getting physical outdoors amidst the fresh air, sunshine, breeze, and negative ions found in nature against the background of blue skies and green foliage boosts mental and emotional wellbeing. When you're indoors, keep well ventilated. Cancer causing gases like formaldehyde and other VOCs (volatile organic compounds) can be found in particleboard furniture and carpets. Spending time outdoors, whether exercising, recreating, or even caring for the lawn and garden, has been linked to greater decreases in tension, anxiety, and depression. More benefits include improved levels of calmness, mental clarity, focus, vitality, and enthusiasm. Don't those sound like prescriptions for health and catalysts for great relationships at home and at work?

In addition, the benefit of increased vitamin D levels as a result of direct exposure to sunlight also contributes to improvements in mood and total overall health. Except for pollution, nuclear fallout, and other hazards, the research certainly isn't telling us to spend more time indoors. Aren't we listening?

I tell my patients that simple things, natural things, can provide wonderful health benefits. Focusing and even just gazing on the changing and varying terrain we see while we're outdoors has been found to stimulate our mind and senses. In an era where people complain of being bored and overwrought with repetition, who doesn't want more stimulation and a varying terrain?

Recreating and working out of doors has also been found to lower levels of cortisol (the body's stress hormone) to a greater degree than the same activities done indoors. This isn't to say we should avoid fitness centers and indoor yoga and martial arts centers, but that the outdoors needs to be where we spend at least some of our time. It's not a bad idea to spend some quality time outdoors every day. Even my grandparents knew this.

By experience, by passed down wisdom, and by positive results, my grandparents knew that it was healthful and joyful to walk to church on Sunday and go for walks after big meals. As immigrants who left their homeland in Italy, they loved getting out of the house and walking their adopted neighborhood in Chicago. They lived through the Depression and some very tough times. They knew enough to take care of their health and wellness. They understood that putting one foot in front of the other enhanced that and gave them a free activity to enjoy. Don't you have some lessons from your ancestors you can draw upon?

My grandparents even ate well. I can't tell you how much I longed for the big family meals that my grandmother and my mother cooked. Being Italian, the meals that bring the fondest memories were the pasta dishes. It always lifted my spirits and I somehow felt my grandmother's and mother's love more acutely as they lovingly prepared my favorite dish—spaghetti and meatballs. Being young and having a high metabolism, I didn't have to worry about carbs back then.

Naturally for my era, those meals were typically followed by some physical movement. I would head outside and eventually locate my friends and we'd be choosing teams for another game of football, baseball, or pickle. Growing up, I would often take a walk with my dad after dinner and I was always active with baseball, wrestling, weight training, and martial arts. Later, in the overly sedentary world that was medical school, I did my utmost to keep moving. After studying for hours on end, I would clear my mind by going out in nature for a walk which helped to recharge my batteries and get me ready for another round of studying.

I regularly advise patients to take up walking to relieve stress and improve digestion. When we were young kids, our elders took us for frequent walks. That was a great way for both of us to spend some recreational time. Besides the benefits to the mind and the heart, the digestive processes are often enhanced when we don't just sit down on the couch right after a meal. Even our stomachs seem to like it when we stroll the sidewalks and paths. And, to help us through our busy schedules and daily challenges, this good digestive health and physical activity is associated with better sleep, often considered the best stress reliever of all.

There are a considerable number of long-term studies that directly associate stress with illnesses, including brain abnormalities, organ dysfunction, and cancer.

What can we do about that? We can de-stress by ensuring some good physical activity with enough sound sleep. Other studies have concluded that enjoyment levels and workout satisfaction are higher for those who train outdoors as opposed to those who train indoors. This suggests that individuals who train outdoors may be more likely to continue to not only engage in a consistent workout regimen due to the mental and emotional benefits, but may also find that their individual workouts last longer, are more focused, and tend to be more fulfilling. How much fulfillment do you feel after ending an entire afternoon flipping channels on the couch?

Sifu Slim makes the point that euphoria is what we all crave. He reminds us the term is derived from the Greek word *euphoros* which means health, a state of wellbeing. Elation is also part of the meaning. This book hits the mark when it enables us to consider the idea that we have an innate drive in seeking health. What you make of that will of course be for you to decide. How you get your health and euphoria is also for you to decide. What Sifu Slim has accomplished in Sedentary Nation is combining the knowledge we've gained from our ancestors stretching back over thousands of years with the latest research on achieving a healthy, active lifestyle. A true wellness approach.

His research enabled him to take a long look at tribal peoples who spent most of their time outdoors, frequently engaged in physical movement—some highly vigorous, some light, and often ending with the term that eludes so many of us today—*Downtime*. I can't disagree with this notion of finding useful answers in the past and I certainly am a big proponent of downtime. We need more of this as we age. That's not to say that today's kids have this in great supply—they're getting increasingly bombarded with sound and imagery, both of which are part of what's driving their decreasing mental and physical health.

You will find this book steeped in history, philosophy, and common sense, yet with creative and actionable steps. A big piece of our modern medical knowledge is based on human history, as well as the millennia-old study of nature, especially botany. As a long-time student of health, I can support the book's emphasis that consistent exposure to natural sunlight may not only improve mood but also help to regulate your circadian rhythm which can help both improve and regulate sleep and boost energy levels.

My suggestion is not to simply take my word for it or Sifu Slim's word for it, but to see how some of this works for you. I like to think of myself as a caring physician who has dedicated a few decades of his life to learning as much as I can about the psychiatric components of human health. I see hundreds of patients per year and these folks all teach me a great deal. As a doctor who practices outdoor living and physical fitness, I may be somewhat different in this way—I normally only suggest lifestyle changes toward practices I myself would do or have done. I know what sedentary lifestyles and indoor living have done to me and I know the antidote, though sometimes elusive, is not that complicated.

Do you want to experience the increased oxygen levels found outdoors among oxygen generating trees and foliage? This can only enhance wellness, workout endurance, and workout recovery. Contrast this with the florescent lighting and air conditioning of most indoor gyms and workout facilities, which may lead to increased fatigue and diminished muscular contractile strength. Working out indoors for extended periods of times on stationary equipment with unchanging environmental stimuli (i.e. staring at the same wall) often increases boredom which can lead to shorter workouts and decreased workout intensity and may result in reducing or eliminating the workout itself.

I suggest that nearly anything's better than perpetually staring at a blank wall. Having said that, we physicians learned long ago that having some outdoor, natural scenes artistically rendered on the clinic's inside walls—and even ceiling … at least that's what some dentists do—furnishes our patients, our staff, and ourselves an inspiration for being out in nature. Actually sitting by a waterfall or a brook outdoors can generate the ultimate in soothing, relaxing, and even engaging experiences. Otherwise we'd never meet up with our sweethearts or write a poem … down by the river.

Just like the water molecules running downstream through the river, we are a collection of individual and interrelated cells. When we are happy, our cells are happy. When we are stressed, so are our cells. Our human cells of course can heal themselves, and the structures they support, and reproduce better with proper diet, exercise, and rest. Vitamin D is not easily obtained from the garden. It's found only in mushrooms, fish oils, and vitamin pills. Without this essential vitamin, the human physiology and brain chemistry deteriorate and we eventually wither away. To those who don't want to waste away like that, get outside a bit every day. Tell your employer and your spouse that your health simply mandates it, and that Dr. Gary prescribed the out of doors for the condition that so many suffer from today—lack of nature and lack of fresh air and sunshine.

In this wonderful life, I have spent decades as a student in sedentary, desk-bound positions, and also as an athlete, a fitness person, a recreational body builder, and martial artist. To some degree, I continue nearly all of the aforementioned activities to this day. Spending substantial amounts of time indoors and at the desk are part of what I must do to keep up my professional pursuits and tend to some of my home life responsibilities. But it will assuredly come as no surprise that long before I started studying medicine, I knew that sitting in confining desks and chairs had noticeable downsides. During long bouts of sedentary postures, invigoration and focus were sometimes hard to come by and sleep and boredom were sometimes easily induced. I certainly wanted to have more joy in my life as well as a happier spinal column.

The remedies were apparent: Get moving and get exercising, outdoors whenever possible. Exercising's benefits, I found, lasted far longer than the post-workout hours. The benefits remained for days. Now in my profession as a practicing physician, I know that what I learned about the outdoors—recreation, exercising, and simple strolls through the neighborhood—are important things to share with patients, especially those whose health histories revealed some outdoor and recreational deficits. Many of my patients also admitted they were sitting too much. Together we determined just where they were missing out on some of the things our grandparents and prior generations had enjoyed just by living their customary way.

My prescription—go back to the olden days. Get off the couch and out from behind the desk, get outside and get physical. Tell the green meadow or local park that Sifu Slim and Dr. Gary sent you.

Gary Casaccio, M.D.
Psychiatrist
Wheaton, Illinois

Preface

"Leave all the afternoon for exercise and recreation,
which are as necessary as reading. I will rather say more necessary
because health is worth more than learning."
—Thomas Jefferson

Granted, among other things, Jefferson was one of America's greatest presidents, principal author of the Declaration of Independence, and fluent in five languages—but what did he really know about fitness and wellbeing that's relevant for life in the 21st century, not the 18th and early 19th?

It turns out almost everything.

For one, his approach to exercise and recreation helped him to live and thrive to the age of 83, which was a well above the average lifespan at that time.

For another, as President Kennedy declared at a White House dinner and reception honoring Nobel Prize winners, "I think this is the most extraordinary collection of talent, of human knowledge, that has ever been gathered together at the White House, with the possible exception of when Thomas Jefferson dined alone." You may have learned about the relationship between exercise and brainpower. Exercise has the capacity to increase the actual size of the hippocampus (part of the memory and spatial navigation center of the brain), which normally shrinks with older age. This shrinking is thought to lead to impaired memory and dementia.

I don't know about you, but I'm all for growing my brain with age and not becoming overly forgetful. I'm sure I'll need to get to my favorite spots around the house and in town. I'll undoubtedly want to recall who that person is in the mantle photo … the young, dashing dude whose arm is around the beautiful woman who looks quite a bit like the woman currently rocking in the chair next to me.

Some folks can't help themselves though; they're bent on busyness. One person who saw Jefferson's opening quote said, "Who's got time for Jefferson's recreation?"

A rebuttal might be, "Do you live to work?"

Chapter 1

Lifestyle in 1910 vs. New Millennium

Question: What are some of the principal similarities and differences between the lifestyle of our forebears in 1910 and our lives today?

Possible Answers: The year 1910, and forward into the next two decades that resulted in the Great Depression, recalls a time of great economic, family, and geopolitical stress. We have suffered matching events in our new millennium's Great Recession. Part of this causes what philosopher Alan Watts called "the anxiety of uncertainty."

How Did the Previous Generations Get Through the Tough Times in the Early Part of the 20th Century?

It wasn't easy but they tallied on. An obvious offshoot of the study of history is how we take away generalities and trends. Which particular trends jump out when we consider the physicality of 1910 versus today?

An observation: Our forebears walked more, moved more, and lifted more. They ate less and sat less. They spent more time with family and no time at the mall. They may have derived more personal and societal fulfillment, and slept better. That's it in a nutshell.

Many of them toiled in exhausting physical jobs. For some, the workday went more than 12 hours and the workweek was seven days. If they wanted to keep their jobs or not fall off the horse, most were asleep within a few short hours of the evening meal. Today, so many stay up late engaged in a myriad of activities: flipping channels, surfing the Net, arguing, and drinking. Some are engaged in what are considered positive endeavors: working with their children, studying, reading, and intimacy.

Staying up late due to being wired or hyper-programmed to consume more information and imagery presents itself as an incredibly significant difference between our ancestors and us. Their sleep was a significant part of their recovery from an almost impossible workweek. They had to have their brain rested and alert for their heavy-duty focus requirements. Handling animals on the farm or handling molten iron meant that one screw up could cost an arm or a life. Food has to keep you nourished. The human engine, especially the brain, requires a steady supply of beneficial calories which are drawn from fat and sugar storage depots in the body.

The rows at the supermarket were entirely different back in the old days. Yes, there were some rows of cans and boxes, but there was much less junk on display. Canning was an ingenious food preservative method that came about as a contest sponsored by France's military between 1795 and 1810. In the early days of canning, the main goal was to preserve food, making it difficult for microorganisms to flourish. Eventually, marketers sought to improve taste, image, and profits. Today we can walk down rows and rows filled with captivating boxes and wrapped goods that excite our taste buds with hints of what's inside. Some of what's inside is the tasty stuff food scientists have spent time concocting. More recently, their formulas have evolved with increasing demands for more nutritious food and less chemicalized food. Green markets have sprouted up, hearkening back to old-school living. But today, it's still quite difficult to find healthful, natural whole-food products at reasonable prices. Even the "healthful cereals" in the healthful markets frequently are laced with cane sugar and other unneeded additives. Would you buy cereal without the sweetened taste? In the old days and even when I was a kid, people added their own sugar or honey. What's so hard about that?

Food purchasing in a store wasn't always self-serve like it is today. Someone on staff once got you what you asked for. That meant experienced shoppers closely examined what they were getting. When they could, they may have rejected the less than appealing offerings. In some instances, vegetables were wrapped in newspaper. You would open what was being handed to you to make sure it was up to snuff ... or sniff.

We know about wars fought over land and oil. There's also a war being fought right in your local supermarket. In a popular videotaped news story, noted food journalist Michael Pollan cruises the isles inside a modern supermarket filled mostly with processed, industrial food. Dr. Pollan is accompanied by Michael Moss, his food industry investigator colleague, who says, "Behind these shelves is the most fiercely competitive industry there is ... They're fighting each other for stomach share."[2] Food and beverage is big business just as oil is big business. These companies are huge spenders on advertising with wine and spirits, fast foods and soft drinks, and sugar and confection leading the way.

A shopping market wants to move its inventory. It wants turnover. Crates and boxes are unloaded by trucks and the goods are fitted into displays on the shelves. Chosen pieces make it to your bag and eventually to your kitchen. It's a constant chain of events we pay for with money and energy. If we sacrifice health in this process, we pay even more. How many affordable quality food stores and fresh-air markets do you have within a short distance from home?

When I lived in France in the 1980s, a buyer had to beware. Returns were not accepted by most food stores. As far as lifestyle and shopping trends, France in the 1980s had a lot in common with the United States in the 1950s or '60s. Smaller, individual stores and fresh-air markets sold meat, bread, fruits, vegetables, and flowers.

The smaller stores were as prevalent as supermarkets and numbers of patrons preferred them to the larger stores. If people could easily walk to the stores or markets, they often did so. In many cases, they pulled along a vertically oriented, collapsable shopping cart for their hauling needs. Neighborhood hardware stores were widely used as compared to more distant and more sizeable home and lumber stores. Some of this "boutique industry" is returning. People do favor convenience and appreciate the local vendor experience which can provide a social component. Increasingly, patrons welcome the social connection to the storeowner and staff, as well as the chance to say hello to neighbors.

The Human Struggle in 1910

Just as is obvious today, this era was comprised of its share of people caught up in the struggle. Outdoing us in sturdiness and physical agility, this generation did more of it with their brawn, tenacity, and cooperation—which has long been nature's way. It would certainly be a step forward for many of us in the new millennium to be half as agile as the majority of our forebears from the last century's turn. And strength, eh hem, when's the last time you or your kids heaved a cumbersome saddle 14 hands up in the air and landed it squarely on the blanket atop a horse's back?

Please take a moment to power off your smartphones because the message here is set to go deep. For the next few days, during your reading time, your voicemail could be changed so your callers will hear: "I'm tied up with Sifu Slim. He cares about me. Talk to ya soon."

It's true, I do care. And, I have a few questions for you.

When's the last time you put a 30-pound rough burlap sack of potatoes over your shoulder, walked it home from the store, and transported it a few flights up to your kitchen, before you peeled them in concert with your family? You once did that so you'd have food for the many mouths in your home—and maybe some food for the neighbors who were hungry? Families and extended families spent a lot of time together. Love, community, and family support go a long way in terms of survival and wellness. Have you hugged and fed someone today? How long has it been since you shared a repast with someone new?

When's the last time you swung your partner in a rhythmic dance like the tango or the mazurka? The harder you work, the more you should play. And I don't mean your thumbs ...

In 1910, there were no TVs or franchised fast-food restaurants.

People consumed potatoes aplenty, but they themselves were rarely couch potatoes—most didn't own a couch. Stuffed, upholstered furniture was a luxury item. Comfort, abundance, and surplus (and the culture of excess) were not established traditions. Heck, the masses didn't even have refrigerators. Meat shops initially handled cold storage using their horse-delivered blocks of ice, and by selling cured or smoked meats. The state of New York alone held 717,000 horses in 1910. Today the West is full of people who eat like a horse. In 1910, it didn't shock anyone to see horsemeat on the menu.

In order to survive, the masses in 1910 needed to work, or stick with their families, or excel at begging. The historical record is full of imagery of workers who were exploited during the industrial age. This was parodied in Chaplin's films like "Modern Times." Those still on the farm had their hardships as well, especially when they were in competition with bigger, more "efficient" farms.

Harsh treatment and the market system led to the formation and membership in labor unions and farmer co-ops. Battles, sometimes with bloodshed and cracked craniums, between management and labor were ongoing. As is the case today, management had influence in high places. But rather than the endless courtroom posturing and arbitration we see today, some of the outcomes were settled old-school style—with clubs wielded by thugs for hire who attacked those in the picket lines or right at their work-camp housing or family residence.

Kids, Take Your Lunch Boxes and Go ... to Work

In 1910, the median number of years of school attended was 8.1 because children were expected to work.[3] Yet most people were not miserable imbeciles, though misery was not hard to find. The economy was growing, but poverty prevailed. The average income was $750 per year; a loaf of bread was 3 cents; monthly rent was a mere $5 to $10. Many workers were first- and second-generation immigrants. Some of these steamship voyagers had given up little or run from ruin to come to America. These immigrant families suffered the power of monopolies, housing barons, and severe competition. Women who fought for the right to vote were ridiculed and beaten for their beliefs. African Americans and other minorities were mistreated and barred from joining labor unions.

The lives of children, especially those in urban areas, were often marked by undernourishment and lack of proper care. Child labor was driven by poverty and sick or injured parents, together with the need for cheap labor. In 1910, child labor laws were infrequently enforced. Subsequently, it was common to see bony or inadequately nourished children toiling long hours for scant rewards.

Besides the recent immigrants, some of these Americans were descendants of longtime residents of the Colonies. Even with severe competition and racism, poverty could thrust people together, encouraging cooperation. The longtime residents and the recent immigrant families somehow made it through. Assistance from families and communities, increasing productivity and standards of living, and a sense of pride helped to make it somehow bearable. Why didn't they give up? It wasn't because they went to a psychologist or a life coach, unless that person also served as grandma. The answer is the same reason many of us don't give up—it's not part of our nature. There was simply no other way.

Few of the residents of 1910—our grandparents and great-grandparents—read Freud or self-help books, went to the psychologist, joined gyms, stayed up late (unless they were on the job or out carousing), ate highly processed junk food, or sat in physical stagnation in chairs, seats, and sofas most of the day, evening, and night. Sitting, especially chair sitting, has been listed as one of the most important drivers of poor health and physical wear in an indoor-oriented, sedentary society.

Many of the body's systems fail to perform normally without physical movement. Fluid builds up and inflammation results from prolonged sitting or standing. You may have noticed your legs aching and swelling on airline flights or when you've been a volunteer standing at a ticket booth. Your body's systems—especially the circulatory system, the lymphatic system, the alimentary system, and the endocrine system—all depend of physical movement to work optimally. You could almost say *to work at all.*

The verb "work" means that something is doing its job, not just keeping you alive. The body is supposed to handle your tasks and empower your mind (and vice versa), and hopefully it allows you not only to survive but also to thrive. That, I suggest, is the most important part of the definition of wellness: the state that results when mind, body, and spirit connect in such a way that we function optimally and are allowed to thrive.

Professional Minimalists

If they only work eight hours per workday, minimalists tend to have more spare time. This can enable them to focus on self, as well as on other people.

In the old days, you had less stuff. The less stuff you had, the more your body was considered important to you, and the more you could focus on it. That's what kids often used to do with free time. They naturally sought to uncover the feats of wonder that could be produced by their minds and anatomy. Roller skating, hopscotch, climbing, double Dutch, stickball, human pyramids, and rolling and tumbling. The working masses of 1910 didn't have huge closets of clothes to concern themselves with or endless boxes of collectibles to organize and maintain. If they were lucky, they had winter clothes, summer clothes, and Sunday clothes. And holes in those were common, though just as commonly mended.

I have long been interested in my New Jersey, German, and mixed-European heritage. My namesake paternal great-grandfather was a musketeer in the German Army from 1869 to 1882. Henry Kreuter immigrated to America in 1890 with his wife, Marie. No one in America knew that he was a good shot back in his military training days, but he did become known as a sharpshooter of his personal spittoon. He was allergic in general and probably allergic to the American flora and spores that were new to him. When he got to America, he lived in Newark, New Jersey—home to a burgeoning chemical and dye plant industry.

Thinking of the smoke stacks along parts of the New Jersey Turnpike can almost produce a 200 mph expulsion of air, also known as a sneeze. Henry walked incessantly both for work and to get around town. He was, as they say, good people and of good cheer. Henry and Marie, not wealthy people, were known to feed the neighborhood in their section of Newark. They were both from neighboring small, farming villages near Alsfeld, Germany.

As a new immigrant to the job mecca of Newark, my great-grandfather wound up working the nightshift for the Erie Lackawanna Railroad. Knowing how cold and clammy my home state's climate can be several months of the year makes the producing of phlegm understandable. He and I were born with sneeze genetics, and there's sometimes not too much one can do about that. But, it's relatively easy to stop the pandemic of sedentary living. You move more and have stretching stations and horizontal bars in the home and workplace. We're so beset with comfort in our homes that this comfort is creating discomfort. Whom do you know who has never experienced hip, neck, or back problems? It's certainly possible Henry the immigrant's generation wouldn't have thought too highly of today's indoor, digitally addicted lifestyles. How could you feed the neighborhood if they won't get off their couches or smartphones?

Some of our ancestors were known to spend a portion of their hard-earned wages on musical instruments. Later, these instruments could be passed down to new generations. Descendants of another side of my family were early arrival American immigrants from England—1635. Perhaps the most talented of the 20th-century progenies was my maternal great-grandfather, George York. He worked as an inventor and master mechanic for Edison Labs, located in West Orange, New Jersey. Besides helping to raise eight children, he still found time to practice and play in a string quintet.

His 1880's mandolin is still in the family—and still works. How long do big screen TVs, last these days? You are assuredly aware they were designed to be unserviceable on purpose. The companies want you to buy them new every so many years. During the years writing this book, a week didn't go by that I didn't see two or three TVs curbside with *free* signs taped to the face. Who can even carry them? What dumpsite even wants their toxicity? Someday in the future, researchers will seek access to Craigslist archives to determine what items people were giving away. Will they be shaking their heads at our wastefulness or, will they look up to it in envy?

Fertility and Virility

Musical instruments last eons longer than smartphones. Because of a number of my habits, I'm considered old school. More than a decade into the new millennium, I still went without a high-end portable communication device. Before I was "forced" to upgrade to a smartphone, I was berated by my contacts for my blocking of text messaging. The cell does serve me well both professionally and socially. It's also producing its share of EMF waves (electromagnetic frequencies from our electrical lines and electrically powered devices) that have been bombarding us since the development of electricity.

Did you know that men who keep them in their pants pockets have noticeably reduced sperm counts? Want children? Invest in a fanny pack but avoid wearing it while seated. Worn in the front, such a pack heats up the groin. Recent reports indicate that male teenagers and young adults have reduced sperm count and libido. Besides smartphones, and excessive visual stimulation, another possible link is the laptop which heats up the temperature and zaps the groin with more EMFs. Most young people I know watch Netflix and other online streaming video lying in bed with the computer on their midsection. This without being separated from body to computer by a plastic cooling plate. Oh, the horror!

Old-school style living was wonderful in this respect: If you wanted to see someone, you got up and made your way to where they might be. Do you feel the urge to interrupt your day to text a loved one or friend on a repeated basis? While I was describing my focus for my writing and workday tasks to a friend, he told me, "So what you're saying is that you don't have text messaging since you don't like the interruptions?"

"Exactly," I replied. "They are invasive. A writer, and anyone with a list of things to accomplish, needs lengthy focus time. A lot of what I do is on hyper-focus time."

"Well," he said. "Your intuition was correct. I just read a report that said each text message takes us three to five minutes to recover from."

"Could be even longer for me," I said. "I'm a grammarian, and I strive to make my emails funny and engaging. I might do the same for texts, and I can type with my two hands on a laptop a lot quicker than I can send texts."

Butt Implants? Don't Tell Great-Great Grandma

The monetary figures are shocking to us today. The 1910 U.S. average of $750 income per year was spent on necessities. This might have included an instrument and a deck of cards, and would likely have included some tobacco and some beer and it was rarely enough to allow for socking away any savings. This type of fiscal paucity would eventually keep your personal savings mostly unaffected by the 1929 stock market crash—you didn't own any stock nor did you have any savings accounts. However, if the Great Depression subjected you to being out of work, you couldn't buy food.

And forget any elective beauty surgery for the working class. Outlandish! If you had a physical abnormality, you probably kept it for life.

If you wanted to change your physique, you might have tried wearing a corset. Consider the modern day rage of butt implants at an unreimbursed $10,000 or so. Can you imagine your great-great grandmother in the hereafter catching wind of that behavior? Even contemplating such an inflated protrusion might cause a crocodile-like rollover in her grave.

A paying job was a big deal. You wanted work. And when you had it, by Jove you wanted to keep it. There was generally little chance to "milk a task" and be a slacker. A slacker on the dock would get an earful from the other longshoremen, if not tossed into the drink.

One Potato, Two Potato, Three Potato Four

A slowpoke on the seamstress assembly line might have a pile of work to complete after her normal shift.

As is customary in the formula for human pitfall, overpopulation and a shorted-sighted outlook were the causes. In Ireland, here's how it is said to have happened. The potato came from South America, through Spain in the 1500s at a time when Ireland held a population of one to two million. This energy-filed tuber or root crop allowed peasants to feed many mouths. In wet soil—aka mud—the potato tends to do well. The population boomed to some 8 million people by 1845, making Ireland one of the mostly densely populated rural regions in the world.

Without foresight or education, and with pressure to feed themselves despite being predominantly relegated to the least-fertile regions, potato peasants in certain regions of Ireland continued to grow potatoes and proliferate. Besides carbohydrate calories, the potato also provides roughage, vitamins, minerals, and even a complete range of amino acids—protein. Though one main crop does not a good diet make, this particular root vegetable was a dietary miracle for feeding a poor population of field workers. A family of four might need to consume some 150 potatoes per day, adding some milk for vitamin D and liquid consistency like we do with breakfast cereal.

Not putting all one's eggs in one basket is an old lesson that is oft-overlooked, except by the airborne fungus that blew onto the fields planted with the Irish Lumper. This staple variety of potato perished in a few seasons, along with approximately one million Irish citizens. Around this time of upheaval, some 20 percent of the Irish left for America in search of a better life. By 1910, more people with Irish blood lived in the United States than in Ireland. Some of them worked as garment workers often in sedentary workstations.

Skilled workers such as garment workers were often seated, which is hard on the anatomy. To circumvent labor laws that were enacted during the industrial period, many laborers, even entire families, wound up working from home around the kitchen table. When you pay employees by the task and quality, not by the hour, there is less need to monitor their work. Such company "employees" who were working from home often received very little sunlight exposure and enjoyed relatively little full-body movement. Though these seated jobs caused repetitive stress and other conditions, these people may not have been as immobile and slouching as today's perpetually computer bound.

As a rule, seated movement was well, more moving in the old days. If the 1910 garment workers sat while working, their hands and arms were in constant movement. At the busy factories, they reached, leaned, and gripped which also activated their lower bodies. It's probable their actions were less biomechanically detrimental than the sedentary desk positions that today result in carpal tunnel, nerve damage, spinal trouble, and disorders of inflammation including atherosclerosis, cancer, and strokes. Think of a concert pianist who really gets into the crescendo, flailing away with powerful keystroking. Compare that to a desk potato whose gaze is focused on the screen, inputting data into QuickBooks or Excel.

Workplace wellness consultant Erik Durak suggests that carpal tunnel was so rare a number of decades back in part because the people were stronger. "When the secretaries went home, they were handling iron pots, buckets, brooms, and kids. Also, remember that the typewriter's carriage return was a separate movement." There is a long list of possibilities on the causes of carpal tunnel in the computer era. Inflammation is prevalent in cultures suffused with stress, poor diets, and sedentary lifestyles. Biomechanically speaking, repetitive stress, especially severe repetition like the digital keyboards, can wreak havoc on the human anatomy.

Try a typewriter sometime. You'll see that the moments spent changing paper and erasing are breaks in the action. Slouching postures generate enough contact pressure to operate a computer keyboard. But with a manual typewriter, the demands for physical strength and proper posture are more significant. An additional observation on typewriter users: They weren't ordinarily coming home and doing more typing. These days, it's not uncommon to see a person work all day on the computer, sit down at a computer at home, and use a smartphone endlessly throughout entire awakened hours.

When I'm involved in a day of writing and research, I may be on the computer more than eight hours. I may have a book in my hands another few hours. Strengthening the arms and hands, taking stretch breaks on the hour, and using good keyboard posture has been the reason for continued functional use of the keyboard. I do wrist exercises by squeezing rolled up grippy gloves (the same kind movers and landscapers use) nearly every day. Sometimes I squeeze them repeatedly during a long jog, or a 20-minute walk around the neighborhood, or for eight minutes during my standing calisthenics.

The proper biomechanics taught to me is to squeeze from pinky to thumb. The hand will close in a punch position while keeping the arms bent at elbows. The punch surface of your fist is straight forward, with first two knuckles up (thumb and index knuckle up). This means the closed palm will face in toward the other hand. Even better, tilt each hand slightly outwardly, thumb and index knuckle about 22 degrees outwardly. That has worked well—no carpal tunnel problems despite lots of computer use.

Squeezing a mushy, rubbery piece of cloth every day may sound a bit much, but, as the saying goes, an ounce of prevention... We have time on our walks to do this. Why not use this time to strengthen key parts of the body? As you can probably tell, exercise persistence is part of my DNA. I also abhor surgery and suffering through recuperation from injury. Though sedentary during my laptop time, I'm creating function through daily exercise and hourly breaks.

Because of my slim stature, you wouldn't necessarily think me strong. It hasn't been for lack of trying, exercise has been a daily pastime since I could climb out of the crib. Some hard work and mental drive has made me fairly adept at bodyweight exercises and functional fitness. But even without much in the way of beefy muscles, I've played a number of strong-person sports—including football. I'm fortunate to have never gone under the knife for any major injury or major biomechanical breakdown.

Good fortune and maintenance exercises has also prevented any carpal tunnel aggravation. I have mangled my hands off and on during my time skiing and doing Brazilian jiu-jitsu. Jiu-jitsu is definitely a contact sport even though the term means "the gentle art."

So, yes, some sports injuries have caused an ample supply of pain, but I have been lucky never to have needed surgery for a sports-related injury or accident.

General Health, 1910 vs. Today

Is it possible the U.S. citizens of 1910 ranked higher in general wellness than we do in the new millennium? That's an interesting question and it might make quite a book. Another way to consider this would be to compare trending averages. Here are some of the negative trends to compare and contrast the life of the workers, aka masses.

1910: impoverished, at times malnourished, overworked, poorly housed, often abused people, who walked a lot, danced when they could, and stuck together for cooperation and survival

vs.

new millennium: overstuffed, sedentary, addicted, channel-flipping, over-medicated, *stressed-out* people, who dance little but watch dancers on TV, and sadly, despite the human need for fellowship, tend to stick more to themselves and often fend for themselves

In any analysis, it's easy to get preoccupied with the short years listed in the 1910 longevity statistics—age 48 for men, 52 for women. These figures are skewed since they included the great number of people who died in childbirth and as children, and from cases of polio and tuberculosis. First, a misnomer to dispel. Besides epidemics like the Spanish Flu of 1917–1918, people weren't dropping like flies in what we now consider middle age. Based on the lifespan tables, if you made it to age 40 back in 1910, you were expected to live on average another 28 years.[4]

Those figures aside, do you think today's headlines—such as the obesity epidemic; rises in autism, asthma, and autoimmune diseases; the medicated nation; the Prozac nation; the fast food nation; the vaccine nation; fragmented families; frankenfoods; lawsuit frenzies; and the 24-hour digital world—are counteracted by some conception of living longer?

I remember one telling moment in my 20s. My then girlfriend and I were on vacation, doing some tourism, driving to a destination with my parents. My girlfriend and I got into an argument about some nonsense in the backseat of their car. My dad tried to calm the turmoil by saying, "Come on you two, life's too short ..." In a moment of lock-and-load honesty, my mom piped in, "No, it's not. It's not too short." That broke us all up and the turmoil was gone.

Do some hope or intend to live longer while being uncomfortable, unwell, on meds, dissatisfied, stressed out, and lonely? All these are common complaints of young and old in our current era. Then there's the infamous gripe parents and teachers hear to no end: "This is boring." There are people who have a fully stocked freezer of their favorite packaged meals, a few hundred cable channels, Internet, the latest hand-held digital devices, and 500 friends on their social media page, yet they complain of being bored out of their minds. We had downtime galore when I was a kid. In the '90s and beyond, adults and the children themselves seem to be over scheduling and overanalyzing everything. If you start out over-scheduled as a kid, where will you end up? Take a break from the rat race and follow your feet and walk somewhere.

Boring, hmm, come to think of it, I have never heard my parents or any of the elders of my family complain of anything being boring. That term's common, popular usage as a complaint seems to have become vogue in the 1980s, along with the surge of sedentism and computers. So, this seems to suggest that "boring" came about with less movement and more "convenience" which then required an overly scheduled life. Hooray for the Franklin "day" Planner. Without that we might have had a needed breather. Who the heck needs a breath anyway?

"Immature is a word boring people use to describe fun people."
—Will Ferrell, comedian, actor. b. 1967, Irvine, Calif.

It's no laugh that the theme of the 1910 masses offers direct parallels to the survival mode many people are experiencing today. Every one of us knows of or has witnessed people who have become destitute due to economic conditions, even those brought on by a health-related problem. How can we get some of the good our struggling ancestors had? How can we thrive while we live in today's denatured culture of good old relationship disharmony, endless information bombardment, mega-sized fitness centers, crowded roads, Big Medicine controlled hospitals and HMOs, mega-supermarkets, and franchised restaurants that too often feature factory-farmed, bastardized food?

Let's work through such questions as we begin the journey

with one vital step. Go take a long stretch break or do an exercise program before reading chapter two. The rush here isn't in the intellect; it's with the physicality of your mindset.

Easy Takeaways

1. The year 1910 was a melting pot of competition and abusive labor practices. But there was also a common trend of families and neighborhoods sticking together. People also generally moved their bodies, tired themselves out, and went to sleep within a few hours after dinner.

2. Today so many stay up late engaged in a myriad of activities: flipping channels, surfing the Net, arguing, drinking, or engaged in what are considered positive endeavors: dialoguing, working with their children, studying, reading, intimacy, etc. Better to rise with the chickens and go to sleep with the chickens. Good sleep and sleep patterns drive happiness, productivity, and wellness.

3. Despite the abuse of a long day with repetitive tasks, we all have to seek out a formula that compensates for the wear and tear and enriches us with movement and realignment of our posture.

4. Old school is something we can learn from—most of our ancestors weren't dimwits and lollygaggers.

Chapter 2

As Denatured as Our Oatmeal

Today most of us are as denatured as our oatmeal.

Where did we sign on to that? What contract or coupon did we receive in the mail?

One could argue that our past spending habits suggest many of us have openly agreed to unhealthful changes. Spending trends and purchasing timelines are easily found on the Web. I spent a good bit of time on the economics and trends in cereal consumption to see how 20th century fads might have impacted our health, budgets, and taste addictions. For me, it was a personal matter.

For almost two years before adolescence, Buc Wheats cereal flakes found their way into my bowl because of the marketing efforts of its maker, not to mention my youthful susceptibility. Eventually, a palpable realization hit me during a horrific opus of high-pitched drilling sounds ... CAVITIES. A long-term caretaker of my teeth, I was stunned how the dentist had just found a few.

He asked me, "What are you eating?"

"Mom's cooking and healthy cereal—Buc Wheats."

He suggested reading the label which of course indicated the popular maple syrup glaze. Mother Nature produces maple syrup, and she stocks it with a number of healthful ingredients—including natural phenols which act as antioxidants; manganese; and zinc—but she's not telling us to slurp it every morning before school. You don't want a daily practice that involves orange juice opening up the tooth surface with acid and then has you sloshing around a sticky, sugary substance like maple syrup glaze which provides long-lasting food for cavity creating bacteria.

A Mouth Walks in the Door

Cereal wasn't on the menu every morning, but the times it was, I learned to choose better options than manufactured sugarized brands. Conscious of being duped by bogus marketing—including models with big white-toothed smiles, together with the sugary taste—I dropped Buc Wheats and other "supposed" health cereals which might have featured sports stars on the box. The new cereal choices became what were the better options like the boxed granola-type cereals available in standard supermarkets. They weren't perfect but they weren't coating my teeth with the lacquer of maple glaze. Result: only a few cavities in the next 10 years. That's a virtual miracle for those of us who eat frequently and have worn braces for extended periods. As kids, we had three meals a day plus snack time. That was a lot of food debris for oral bacteria to enjoy.

A supermarket patron has to read labels, look things up, and listen to honest and informed health experts. An observant practitioner of preventive dentistry has the time and ability to discern and listen to many things about your life and health: dental caries, stress markers, your current family and relationship news, and of course your level of health and fitness. They see you for much longer appointments than the typical medical doctor. You could start by asking a dentist some health questions. One dentist shared, "Some think we see a mouth walking in the door. We're trained to see a whole person walking in."

Where's the Nature?

That's one of my catch phrases.

If you showed me a lifestyle of indoor living, my response might be: "Where's the nature?"

You show me a person who only exercises or recreates in a gym, I might respond: "Where's the nature?"

Would you sign a petition if it said, "Are you in favor of promoting more natural living"?

Historically, living meant covering distances on foot, often carrying things like food, water, and hunting and gathering implements.

Today, outdoor aficionados take up cross-country backpacking or exercising in a park while others see these as anachronistic expressions of aberrant behavior we can credit to "those people who don't have our busy schedules." The hands of time know we are diurnal by nature. Up with the sun, down sometime after the sunset. Outside during the day, inside a structure at night. When we forget that, and we don't even get a lunch break out of doors, we omit a crucial step toward being true to our nature. This causes us to suffer. You may have heard people suffering of seasonal affective disorder. By golly, we all suffer when we don't get enough natural light and exposure to the sun. Denatured, indoor living, and sedentism—these are all part of unnatural living. Today's kids know that. Just ask them. Try this with a suburban or city kid.

"Hey, young fellah. Yeah, you with the iPhone and earplugs. I have a question for you. You ever go to the country, pet a cow, go hiking on a trail, be away from cell phone coverage?"

I have personally asked scores of young people that very question. Nary a one has said they didn't dig that rural experience. One person even recalled mistakenly setting her foot down in a cow pattie.

I've also asked those who have played Monopoly: "Which is more fun, World of Warcraft (an online fantasy multiplayer video game) or some other computer game played from your bedroom, or Monopoly in person with a group of friends?"

Monopoly wins nearly every time but I have yet to ask that question at a video-gamers' conference.

I spent almost over two decades living in or near the SF Bay Area, a region abounding with hiking trails, beaches, and parks. It's also packed with some 7.5 million inhabitants plus visitors—nine million per annum are said to visit the Golden Gate Bridge. The hiking trailhead parking lots fill up quickly on weekends and holidays but they're not being used by the majority of the inhabitants. As far as hiking goes, the same people are coming back to hike and walk. The homebodies aren't coming out.

Parks, trails, and most things outdoors often seem to be on the modern list of no-fly zones for couch potatoes parked on expansive sectionals and at office desks.

The step indoors and the move away from nature did not begin yesterday. If sustainable farming is the last time we were connected to the outdoors for most of the day, most Westerners left those particular farms several generations ago. Anthropological records—mostly seeds and coprolites (aka poop)—suggest agriculture has been with some geographical regions for about 12,000 years. In many places, the move to modernize was a distant, slow-moving revolution. When it came, it often ushered in an authoritarian hierarchical society with plenty of favoritism. More local and stored food translated to more kids per woman per decade as opposed to hunter-gatherers who tended to have far fewer children.

Hierarchy meant there were the order givers, of course bodyguards to protect their interests, and lowly exhausted workers, toiling in the fields getting bitten by flies, bees, and mosquitoes. How long would you want to stay at that sort of smelly and exhausting existence? Since they were strong and at times expendable, the workers could be used for battle against bands of rivals. And many times the lowly workers were glad to exchange a hoe for a sword and a chance to change up their struggle. At least it was a new field of battle.

The movement away from hunting and gathering toward raising animals and sowing crops was not a direct line. Hunting and gathering, as long as there were things to hunt and gather, continued on despite the rise of agriculture. Agricultural practices of seeding, tending, and picking often advanced slowly in some cultures—predominantly those with efficient access to sufficient calories. But when farming, weather, and workers enjoyed favor and efficiency, the populations exploded, as witnessed in the time leading up to the Irish Famine.

Plant It and People Will Come

Many populations were generally content with hunting and

gathering. Some cultures—especially those from the arctic, desert, woodlands, and jungles—were obviously not always set up with open fields and temperate climates to provide lands for the Agricultural Revolution. But arid soil could be irrigated, trees could be cut down, and rich jungle soil planted with food and pastures.

All of this development of structuralized farming terrain and buildings requires mechanical energy output, by man or draft animal. With the advent of fuel oil, the world population boomed. Sustainability activist Paul Chefurka takes up the economic and population growth spurt and production curve called Peak Oil. To Chefurka, and countless others, oil dependency remains "the elephant in the room." This theory suggests that the overpopulated world has over extracted oil. The fallout can only be a dearth of oil and resultant population decline. When man began producing new fuel-based power, food production fueled an exponential increase in population. Overpopulation theorists want the masses to change their ways before there's a great awakening that we're out of water. Satellites are already showing the dry hot spots around the globe in places of high population or high agricultural production. Most of the known aquifers are in peril. What does that mean for us ... and our descendants?

Expiration Dates of Humans

Cultures of historic hunting and gathering still exist today but make up far less than 1 percent of today's world population. Living off boxed food exists on a plane far away from living off the land. In the spatial plane of the modernistic West, we have succumbed to the draw of image and taste. Far too many of us buy based on custom, convenience, and an artful label. Profiteering has us digging into boxes for food that as a general rule has been distance shipped either frozen or dried, and potentially laced with preservatives. Note the lengthy expiration dates printed on the sides of some of those containers. A significant percentage of all processed food and seasonings is wheat based or corn based, or contains ingredients derived from these king crops. Wheat is grown differently than in prior centuries and the wheat is hybridized. Corn is hybridized and GMO.

People's expiration dates may be considered longer than they've been in generations—agreed. But, today, as far as quality of life is concerned, we're often fried, wired, and tired.* Do you think we're a bit overwhelmed by convenience? Maintaining 20 contraptions of convenience isn't all that convenient. Do I hear 30, 50, 100?

Recently I purchased a replacement water pump for my sweetheart's garden fountain. That plastic-coated motor died in four months. The receipt lost, there was no reprieve from the hardware store (one hour of total time), and none after being on hold with the manufacturer. Two total pump hours now spent, I stuck the pump in my car. Amazingly, one last test revealed the pump had undergone some form of resurrection. It worked in a bucket test. Now to reinstall it and try it some more. You undoubtedly have your own pump-ish stories. Think back. When was the last time you were on hold for tech support? When was the last time you had to dig for a receipt and drive an extended distance to deal with

---

* Any person with an argument has to be careful about their assumptions, what they would like to believe. I have done my homework, made my observations, tested their validity, and have put the story of sedentary lifestyles in as artful a way as I can. I welcome your insight and comments on these questions, which you can deliver via the blog at *SedentaryNation.com*

the return of an item?

It seems to take a substantial amount of time, energy, and money to keep phones, computers, and autos functioning properly. Then there's the home, the body, the relationship, the family, the spirit ...

Attempts to satisfy such needs are commonly squeezed in after a long day at work. How does this lifestyle compare with the hunter-gatherers? Going far back in time, were daily chores and wellness pursuits handled substantially differently from how we live today? Were the hunter-gatherers able to care for their bodies and minds, and many of the remaining needs of the tribe, all in a normal day of movement and activity? Did they have downtime?

The downtime statistic is a point of contention among some anthropological scholars. I'm fine with the contention. "It's all good," as the saying goes. I believe the more downtime supposition may be a bit more accurate and enduring than many other historic guesses.

When at peace and when they had access to sufficient, long-lasting calories, or enjoyed steady success accessing the quicker burning food, tribal cultures tended to enjoy downtime. For one thing, they weren't hoarders. Minimalism generally spells more downtime. A look into the written accounts of tribal life of the Indians of North America suggests a history of uneasy periods with marauding tribes, not to mention the pressures of the invading white Europeans. Downtime interrupted by savage killing and looting is something those of us who have always lived in a peaceful zone have never experienced first hand.

That said, how many of us take up downtime outdoors in a quiet way? When was the last time you enjoyed a peaceful hour at sunrise? When was the last time you saw young people enjoying laughter-filled, digital-free, outdoor time at sunset? When was the last time you and your friends and family, aka your tribe, shared a peaceful, worry-free moment watching the free play of youngsters at anytime? How often do you allow yourself to go a bit expressively wild? If you do go wild, are you able to do it without being on any mood-altering substances?

Letting it out, whatever "it" is, is a good thing.

In the Wild and In the Cell

A look at wildness and natural versus denatured living takes some doing. What if we considered animals? Might this help compare people in today's world to people who live or lived close to nature? Next time you are able, watch wild animals doing what they do as they live in their natural habitats. Also watch wild animals that are confined in man-made surroundings. See how monkeys and lions in zoos spend their time. Draw your own conclusions from there. Consider their movement and their bored, even frustrated looks. Interestingly, monkeys, even in zoos, don't sit still for very long. Since their movement is significant, they burn the same number of calories per day as monkeys in the wild.

Here's a concise attempt to explain a very general picture. People in today's world attempt to control their surroundings and each other in respect to spatial, nutritive, financial, and entertainment desires and needs. They are quite capable of eating and drinking themselves into total human expansion and death. Some people are adept at positioning themselves higher up so others can do the grunt work. Despite hierarchies, most native peoples generally shared in the work, teaming up for the various individual and tribal needs. Compared to us, they spent more time on the basic needs of food, shelter, family, and downtime. To have the time to watch life is to enjoy it.

"If we have not quiet in our minds, outward comfort will do no more for us than a golden slipper on a gouty foot."
—John Bunyan, Christian preacher,
author of "The Pilgrim's Progress" (1628 Elstow,
Bedfordshire, England – 1688, London, England)

Today's domesticated animals have a lot of time on their hands. Those unable to roam have so little to do. As they wait for our next inspiration to provide their bale of hay, many of our domesticated, non-roaming animals just have to deal with us. Those we eat tend to be treated poorly; those we own as pets and see every day generally get treated better. Cats and dogs, and other house pets that live with us, wind up in our direct visual path. We tend to treat them better than those in the back pen. Think of a dog that is penned in a dog run far out back. He's left more on his own than the housedog.

How do the lives of wolves in the wild compare to wolves in a zoo? Would you imagine them happier hunting for their food and roaming nature's hilltops, or sitting around in a concrete zoo, eating mostly the same man-made or man-issued slop, pooping in the same corner of their cells for 15 years?

Some of us observe how inherently fragile is the balance of nature. If man were a proper part of this balance, he wouldn't be causing so much damage to it. Man realizes very quickly how devastation occurs. A friend of mine once decided to save some garbage space by dumping the contents of a bag of water-softening salt on a small corner of his back lawn. The area was still bleached out and dead several years later. He basically created his own dried out version of the Salton Sea.

The natural environment is designed to rejuvenate within the framework of normal patterns of nature. A significant number of man-made products are not. Happily, we are making more and more compostable products. While you consider our place in nature and nature's inherent majesty, consider this question. Is there anything man-made that will continue working with minimal upkeep and endure long enough to outlast the lifespan of a giant sequoia? I can't think of anything. Can you? One piece of human achievement that will outlast an ancient tree is the half-life of toxic radiation.

Let's jump back to animals and their physical movement.

Animals in the wild are practiced in the art of living naturally. Semi-active house cats aren't so bad either. From house cats and cats in the wild that are successful in their acquisition of food, water, and shelter, we learn that downtime and a few stretches and some clawing sessions (a cat's total body workout) seem to work miracles. Now for a big leap in comparisons. Would you agree that most people are wired more like the dog breeds that require much more in the way of physical activity? They get antsy, flabby, and rickety if they don't do some purposeful movement.

Why Do Animals in the Wild Move So Graciously?

Answers that top the list are:
1. They live in their natural surroundings.
2. They eat what they're supposed to eat.
3. They move in efficient ways.
4. They move frequently.

Stick a highly active dog breed like a Jack Russell terrier in a confined space with infrequent opportunities to go out for walks and see what you get. Take a six-month-old black Lab from his farm life and send him to live with someone who rarely leaves a downtown studio apartment and see how the dog does. Those two examples drive home the idea that movement is a positive and sedentism is a negative. In the wild, if you don't move efficiently, your chances of survival are severely compromised. In drywall captivity, especially with clutter and dust, your chances of going batty are excellent.

Some of you may be wired more like house cats. That's fine if that is truly the case. But if you were like that as kids in the pre-1970's West, I'd wager you were part of a very small minority. Most of the people I have talked to and grew up with were ready to run and play like an unleashed Labrador retriever or a climbing, roaming cat. Our biochemistry used to say go; whereas, for many today it seems to say no.

Whatever your beginnings, where are you now?

What do you think about how we look and how we carry ourselves? And what we do with our time at work and at home? Is it possible that we have less zip and more melancholy than our ancestors in the Great Depression? How does our will to survive and thrive compare with those of the last plague or Ice Age?

Drywall forms the caves so many of us wind up loathing yet rarely leave. Drywall doesn't protect us from errant or intended bullets, but it does have a way of "protecting" us from outside air, nature, and vitamin D production from the sun. When we do venture out, vehicles, scooters, lifts, and escalators are there to assist us. Is this notion of a sedentary lifestyle part of a safety mechanism?

These are important points you can test for yourself.

What "out there" are some of you so afraid of? What keeps you almost perpetually walled up inside? What are you protecting yourself from? Why the fear? How can you move beyond this fear? If not fear, then why the acceptance of a static state? Why the lethargy?

Fear or Comfort?

It's understandable that people don't want bugs buzzing around them. It makes sense that we want warm beds devoid of slithering reptiles. But why don't some of us venture outside even for a stroll?

Then there is the growing trend of using mobility scooters. Mobility scooters have both positive and negative sides. One negative side is that not everyone who uses them should be using them. One physician I spoke with told me that he is deluged by growing numbers of people who want to get prescriptions for mobility scooters so insurance or social programs will pay for them.

What is this all about? Do some of those who have devices to assist locomotion suffer an uncontrollable fear? Will they be exposed to other's judgment and ridicule? What happened to canes and walkers? Suppose a man falls on the street or in the store. Will no one come to his aid? Some of this psychological reflection may reveal why so many are afraid to take the risk of leaving their four walls or protected mobility devices. Do these gifts of technology give disabled people (including the morbidly obese) a temporary competitive advantage over those who can walk? Of course, this isn't to cast aspersion on people with disabilities, but to examine why we have gravitated to devices of locomotion.

Picture a scene that could almost be part of a prequel to "WALL-E," the Academy Award-winning Disney/Pixar movie of

2008. In that film, Earth has been abandoned and left behind as a massive garbage dump of trash and junk food. The remaining obese earthlings are now conveyed everywhere they go within a huge spaceship because they long ago lost the use of their legs from atrophy, overeating, and gaming (plugged into video programming) rather than experiencing a historically real life of physical activity.

A precursor scene unfolds today. What we count as exercise is only a slow stroll through an interior landscape, the super mall, which taxes the energy of the throngs, who, despite the regular spike from the supersized coffee, soda, or energy drink that dangles in the hand, are game only for nearly any artificial contrivance.

Making it even worse, some of us walk around as if in a zone, consuming whatever our credit can cover with a swipe of a magnetized card that tracks our every purchase and may even be generating emails and text messages to keep us in line and in the new self-service lines, or returning to the checkout lines.

Does this ring true to how things are going these days? How do we compare our endless consumption of goods and fads to the truly sustainable lifestyles of those who live more on laughter, music, movement, and simplicity? How fair is the adage, "different strokes for different folks," if or when we run out of water and arable land?*

Does the presence of fast-food wrappers on our walkways bother you? Are the ubiquitous discarded plastic bottles harmful to critters in the wild? Does it generate any hostility when so many teachers and medical clinicians are grossly unfit—not practicing

---

* Arable means you can grow things in it. To expand a mind, it has to be used. Learning 300 new words per year is 3,000 in 10 years. One charge is to guard against the sedentary nature of our intellect.

good health—yet want us to follow their advice for living? Even the masters have to bow out on some things. My years in martial arts have taught me there are a number of so-called masters who are devoid of well-rounded adherence to healthful living. They can only caution their students with statements like, "Do as I say, not as I do."

Signing on to the social contract means we're not supposed to screw things up and burden society.

Then there's the all-important obedience to the media-imposed culture, you know, looking a certain way and acting according to what is in vogue.

The laws of nature never change, and societies have destroyed themselves and their surroundings before. Easter Island once had trees, and some researchers posit that without trees the islanders perished. The mighty Roman Empire disintegrated in gluttony, illness, disrepair, and corruption.

Is it okay to break the laws of nature but abide by the laws of social acceptance?

Do You Need to Pay Monthly Dues Or Just Move Your Anatomy?

That brings us to the gym. Why do we need them?

Moneymaking—together with a potential answer to inactivity, unwellness, and obesity—has a vast number of the modern exercisers working out indoors. We're sold on the idea that the gym is where we're supposed to fill up our lungs, sweat to the booming beats, and expend calories and hard-earned pay. All this while we work out in an ultra-controlled environment, customarily devoid of any sense of natural setting. Everything these days is done with marketing, new machines, and the almighty dollar in mind.

Bah, humbug to most of that. The best gym I have ever found is the human body itself. Dexterity and grace don't seem a byproduct of many of the machines in the gym. But grace does come from moving the body.

Not everyone goes to the gym for overload training, also known as resistance training. The gym has many wonderful offerings. But I will say this about overload training—it normally produces larger muscles and stiffness simultaneously. You rarely meet fit and well people who happen to suffer an injury doing calisthenics or doing ballroom dancing. But you do hear talk of those who have "popped something" heaving weights, or "pulled something" on a weighted machine or doing a heavy rep on free weights. By its very nature, overload training produces its share of muscle pain and joint stiffness.

That's not to say that weight training doesn't have substantial musculoskeletal benefits. But in a desk-bound, couch-bound, sedentary society of aging people, the place to start is not with building bulk or large-muscle-group strength, but rather with actual physical movement. Can you see that dancing, climbing, crawling, hiking, and biking are forms of movement; whereas weights and resistance machines are generally not getting the body covering any distance? Is your goal to remain in the same place—sedentary—while you put on muscle and bone density with resistance training? If so, how about your posture, and the movement capacity of your body? Here are some simple tests for both exercise routines and sedentary activities. As you do your program of exercise, are your joints making noises? Are you in prolonged discomfort during or afterwards? The functionality for sedentary positions is also easy to test. When you sit or stand for extended periods, do you feel out of balance or achy? For example, does one hip click or cramp up? If you are an exercise person and are doing well with these functionality tests, you may be doing fine with the functionality part of your program.

Last night at a dinner gathering, a former resident of Los Angeles remarked, "People in L.A. drive 30 minutes through traffic to get to work, sit in a cubicle all day, drive home through worse traffic, and then step on their treadmill to walk or run for 30 minutes. Sounds a bit daft, doesn't it?"

What about an outdoor experience? Do you want to hang out in a gym, garage, or basement for 60 years? That's as denatured as it gets.

Get yourself tested for biomechanical strength. If your functionality tests poorly, you'll probably be counseled to build functionality with training like Pilates, and other forms of functional movement exercises. For people who don't need weight loss, most personal trainers have switched from the *bigger, faster, stronger* modality of training to starting with functional training and core training. In this way, the program is designed so the physical structure can better hold itself together. This means the body will better be able to handle physical stress and move with enhanced balance and stability. This directly translates to fewer injuries and improved recovery from injury. This balances the human anatomy. Functional training encompasses exercises similar to yoga and Pilates. Think of the plank and the physio ball (aka exercise ball) exercises. The first time I tried to balance kneeling on a physio ball, I was a dud. Three times later I was able to do it with some grace. It's been the rage of our performance athletes for some two decades. If proper techniques are used, this functional exercise on an inflatable ball builds strength and balance, thus increasing performance.

The payoff for functional fitness is better posture, structural strength, and rehabilitation for injury and areas of weakness. Once you realign your body and test well for functional fitness, the modality of bigger, faster, stronger training can be added. Here's the kicker. Almost no one is able to do the bigger, faster, stronger exercise regimen for a lifetime. Most who try to keep this up, stop exercising completely at some point—usually from injury or the loss of oomph and skill that comes with age. Tennis legend Jimmy Connors was known to play every point like it was match point. Talk about using your focus and force to its fullest. Besides being one of the first great pros to take the ball on the rise, his seemingly endless mental endurance was what carried him through to the records over more than three decades of high-level tennis competition. He segued to golf in his 50s and saves his former go-for-broke physical oomph for other things. His contemporary Bjorn Borg retired from the pro circuit at age 26. His willingness to subject himself to travelling every week or two, remaining at such a high level of physical and emotional preparedness, was over. The moral of the story: Set your course for the aging process as these two icons were able to do. Don't overdo things; use your oomph wisely so you'll have it later in life.

During my five decades of daily exercise, I made the conclusion that daily movement activities should provide some regular outdoor recreation. Getting outside provided the high and the release, which may help us continue doing movement exercises for a lifetime. Outdoor living is in sync with our evolutionary programming. When we do it, we want to do more of it. It's an attraction that's undeniable. Nature itself helps us release endorphins, and it draws us in and reprograms us for wellness. That said, I understand people who have to handle extreme temperatures. In Florida, you can get up early and get outside before the sun. In a cold winter area, you have to bundle up or exercise when it's not overbearing.

Far from the soldiering toil of my great-grandfather, I've had memorable physical workouts in harsher weather. To get outdoors, I've donned a one-piece ski suit in places like Switzerland and Colorado. I've even tromped through piles of snow to use kids' playground climbing bars for chin-ups as the snow was falling. It's tough to beat the bond of gloves adhering to sticky snow. Chin-ups and push-ups do wonders for our strength, posture, and overall health. Movements like these can be done for a lifetime, modifying the movements to make them easier as one needs to. For example, performing push-ups against a low wall or the back of a couch or park bench substantially reduces the weight we bear. For easier chin-ups, string a rope or long martial arts belt over a vertical bar or tree branch and then lean back like you're windsurfing. This allows you to do modified chin-ups and pull-ups as you still keep your feet grounded to the Earth. Nearly everyone can easily pull the load of their reduced body weight. This is very low impact and substantially reduces any chance of muscle pulls in a fit person. Unfit people should start with a program that suits their current level of health and fitness.

If wellness is the goal, you may agree that not doing these types of weight-bearing exercises is a royal downer. Avoiding full body exercise completely is nearly a guaranteed recipe for a sore, stiff, and dysfunctional body. Atrophy sets in very quickly in most of us. And, continued inactivity builds an unhealthful body that deteriorates at an accelerated rate. Who wants that?

People who develop such a lifetime program and work on maintenance fitness or recreational fitness, as opposed to transformational fitness, have a much easier time with physical and mental wellness. Transformation means you want to change your physique. That's fine to a point—as long as you are true to your own physical structure. Ectomorphs, like me, Gilligan, Kate Moss, Whitney Houston, and Bruce Lee gain mostly pain and frustration, not substantially larger muscles, when they try to build bulk on their slim frames. Part of Bruce's incredible muscle building program included some heavy overload training. Unfortunately he wound up breaking his back. Once I had heard that he was doing a leaning over exercise called good-mornings. Bruce's close friend, co-actor, and training partner, Bob Wall, cancelled that notion. During an interview with Bob for my second volume of The Aging Athlete Project, Bob shared that Bruce injured his vertebrae doing squats. Endomorphs, like the rounder football linemen, tend have a difficult time getting slim except when they become ill, suffer addiction, or become aged.

Mesomorphs like Schwarzenegger, Fabio, Mike Tyson, Madonna, Serena Williams, and Beyoncé can put on fat and muscle weight with relative ease. Many mesomorphs have told me they began working out with weights in high school, concluded puberty, started to put on size, and were able to double their bench press max around the years from age 18 to 22.

Mesos can also get more streamlined with diet and exercise. For example, during the filming of Conan, Schwarzenegger is said to have dropped a few dozen pounds to simulate starvation. In the film, Conan is left tied to a tree to die a warrior's death.

For those of you who have simply gotten unfit, any change you wish to make may not be so easy. But, there's good news for some of you. If you were fit once, the body remembers this. This easier bounce back proposition is known as muscle memory. The problem is often mindset. If you keep thinking that going to the gym is what you need to "get back in shape," or to "stay in shape," you may be in for a much tougher time with respect to your physical wellness. I know people who used to love the gym. Essentially, it was their hangout. Now, many of these former gym rats I'm referring to are paunchy people who have put on an additional 40 or 120 pounds of blubber ... that they paid for at the food and beverage stores.

For some of these people, they can't go back to the gym— many seemingly never want to set foot in a gym again. It's sometimes a question of embarrassment. They don't want to prove to themselves how weak, unfit, and uncoordinated they are compared to their former selves. Former high performance aging athletes have shared this exact observation with me. They did their time of intense training and now they're done with that phase of life. You can read about this topic in my book "The Aging Athlete."

Do You Wanna Step Outside?

Here's a bit of my personal fitness history.

Let's begin at age 29 which spelled a big departure from my heavy-duty indoor training. *Après* one final, cardio-funk aerobics class, an additional hour on free weights and machines, and a shower, I walked out of an indoor mega-gym. This was in 1992 and indoor workouts were a regular pastime of mine. Often I was at the big gym three or four times per week, doing varied and professionally planned workouts and aerobics classes. As Popeye is known to say, "That's all I could stands, I can't stands n'more!"

The other days of the week, I was outdoors doing fitness or sports after work. Since the outdoors seemed more akin to what would provide the most benefit at the time, the decision was eventually made to perform the majority of the workouts outside. The working world had me spending most of my daylight hours in offices. More and more, I began longing for outdoor recreating.

A preferred regimen was calling, and this new deal would allow spending more fitness and recreation time out in nature. You know, go natural. This proved to be a big boost for the health of my psyche, mindset, and lungs. Outdoors meant nature, as well as vitamin D—with benefits including stress relief, bone and tooth health, disease prevention, and a list of benefits too numerous to mention. The outdoors delivered instant freedom. I wanted to be a kid again, running naturally, with freeness of form and wind in the hair. I wanted to see things far off in the distance and run to them. I wanted to stick my feet in the river water at the end of my run. Living in a suburban setting, this came to me with ferocity in 1992, as an epiphany, a virtual call of the wild.

Stepping outside of drywall made me appreciate nature and expect more in the way of continued efforts to clean it of man-made debris, and rally a mindset to preserve it.

Treat the earth well.
It was not given to you by your parents,
it was loaned to you by your children.
We do not inherit the Earth from our Ancestors,
we borrow it from our Children.
—Ancient American Indian Proverb

Take Time for Yourself

You are the only you you've got.

Being able to realize where your imbalances lie is an awareness skill that needs to be both acquired and acted upon. That's always been a personal driving interest—creating balance and harmony in the pie chart of my interests, responsibilities, and actions. Of course failure has occurred on repeated attempts.

Bouncing your concerns off comrades and confreres often helps flesh such things out. What came out was that spending so much time indoors, especially when living at the time in Sacramento—a city that boasts more than 300 days per year of sunshine—seemed a bit daft. It took me several years of what finally culminated in indoor delirium to realize that. To be fair, the greater indoors of fitness had delivered plenty of good times, following the popping moves of my upbeat aerobics instructors and enjoying camaraderie with fellow gym members. I honor those good times as I continue to embrace the freshness of the outdoors.

Since that time I have been exercising more efficiently, not less. My energy increased since my system was doing far less in the way of post-workout muscle repair now that overload training had mostly been dropped. Today I still overload biceps, forearms, and shoulders with dumbbells one or two times per week. But in 1992, when I walked out of the gym, instead of stiffness and joint pain, now it was about being fit and functional. My weight dropped two pounds, but my fluidity of movement developed markedly. My push-up max reps went from 30 to 65. Before this, I did early-morning workouts two times per week. Now I did them daily. This would eventually allow me to take up martial arts a few times per week in the evening. That was probably the best bonus of all. When others were dropping "kid stuff" and gravitating to the gym, I was recreating outdoors in the morning and grappling with jiu-jitsu training partners later in the day.

Interspersed for more than a decade, my time with weights and machines had frequently kept me too stiff to do justice to the smoother skill sports of golf and tennis. When I switched to biomechanically functional fitness, the smoothness came back instantly.

I do know folks who do well and gain a lot from the gym. The big question I have is this: How many people can do four to five gym workouts per week for a lifetime? Maybe some only need one or two sessions per week to get what they're after. Being someone who has too frequently sat on his duff at a work computer, daily physical movement has been of great relief. If The Great Indoors works better for your fitness, keep it up. But make sure to get outside for walks, to relax, or to push that stroller. Make sure you connect with nature and get some fresh air and sunshine. When you can, kick your shoes off and get grounded to the Earth.

Last night, I went to a fundraiser kickoff party for a physical movement and dance program for seniors who have mental disabilities. The host was their movement instructor. For over two decades, she has been booked solid by the senior centers since the seniors love this and respond to it. The majority of the attendees to the garden party were within a decade or two of being the same age as the seniors shown in the photos. Dancing outdoors on a portable dance floor made our evening about movement as much as camaraderie and enjoying the food and refreshments. During the break for announcements, the host said her goal was to create *a world dance party* where the entire world could dance outside and express themselves. I vote for that. Are you in?

The Banes of Modern Health

Movement is a good, sedentism is not. Anyone who has seen bedsores or people trapped in a cubicle or ticket booth can visualize the negatives of sedentism. What else should we concentrate on besides movement? Much of the fashionable literature decries diets of high sugar and highly processed foods. Among the other sides of an unbalanced lifestyle are obviously high stress, improper rest, and the two-edged sword of overwork and lack of downtime. Predisposition to problems and disease due to genetics, a hard life, and even karma are other points to consider.

We've all got our baggage.

How do you intervene to change the course of some of these negatives?

You Begin the Program of Self-Mastery

Part of this approach considers the spirit and intentions. Other steps attempt to figure out how to repair the engine and body and then maintain it in its working state. Self-mastery requires a daily awareness, a push, and an acceptance. The golden rule here is to not cause harm as you push yourself to new accomplishments. The definition for self-mastery is unbounded. You can both fixate on certain goals, and take a broad look at how you fit in to the world and your soulful existence.

High Intensity, Heavy Duty Training

Back in time there were Spartans and other warriors whose training was so hard that dying during the drills was a realistic possibility. Properly hitting rocks with hammers, and breaking wood with the bare hands builds stronger bones. African tribes had coming-of-age rituals of fighting with staffs. Pitted against much stronger and experienced warriors, the adolescent boys received on onslaught of smacks to the head and body. Someday they would be able to repeat the exercise as deliverers of the smacks. Many will recall the *no pain, no gain* motto of the 1980s that people got to hear every time they popped in a Jane Fonda aerobics video. This language of this catch phrase goes back in time to Ben Franklin's writing, an earlier English poem by Robert Herrick, and an ancient Hebrew text called Perkei Avot. The notion that anything good comes from hard work is not new to the story of humanity.

As far as training the body goes, very few people seem geared to be do repeated, high intensity/heavy duty physical training forever. For many people, these programs are excessive and will result in breakdown or simply an unwillingness to continue. High intensity/heavy duty means things like boot-camp style training, mud runs, sprinting sports, Olympic weightlifting, and tire flipping. While they are wonderful things for some people to take part in, for most of us, they are not maintainable. Also, high intensity/heavy duty programs should not be confused with smoother activities like maintenance fitness training, as well as lifetime sports including tennis, dancing, hiking, biking, ping pong, and no-motorized-cart/ walking golf. Sports educators have been teaching about lifetime sports for several decades. Why? Because they know kids won't be playing competitive football and soccer forever. The idea is to learn physical things you can take up for a lifetime.

In my 50s, I still do periodic high intensity/heavy duty training by doing tire flipping, crawling, sprint swimming, and sprinting uphill. I don't, however, flip tires or crawl like it's a race. The form has to be true and the exercises have to be done with attentiveness to our healthful limitations. The uphill sprinting is known as high intensity interval training. It's one of the most challenging physical activities I do. But for me, it's easier than sitting on an airplane for five hours.

If you are fit and wish to challenge your system with some short bursts that will also mellow you out, try uphill interval sprints. Try the sprints after a good session of floor exercises and stretching: I typically do 45 minutes or one hour of functional training (more on this later) and core exercises before embarking on the sprints up an incline. In my 20s, I was able to do these sprints at full throttle after a short warm-up jog. If your form begins to fail, stop right there and just walk or jog the rest of the way. Injury prevention comes with listening to the rational mind, not the ego or the excessive coach. Are you aware how hard it is to live with degeneration of the human body, especially the injuries caused by unreasonable behavior, poor preparation, or the ego? Are you aware how hard healing becomes for most of us later on in the aging process. As I write this, a pre-cramp twinge in the left hamstring prompts me to get up and do some stretching. This morning, I did one extra sprint up the grassy knoll.

Some of you may have kids who are doing high intensity training—maybe in school sports or junior lifeguard training. With proper breaks and changes in the weekly training, you may have watched two things happen. One, those kids make incredible gains. Two, they tend to feel super human. A third thing you may have witnessed is a pulled muscle or torn ligament. Injuries have a way of taking an athlete down to a hobble in one regrettable moment. Kids pull muscles and sprain ankles just by being physical kids.

Ask any competitive athlete or recreational weekend warrior how many times they've been on crutches? I can remember four times specifically. Two of those were ghastly ligament tears.

No one wants to come down from a super human outlook and performance level. The truth is, nearly everyone comes down. Charley French, age 88, is a champion triathlete featured in book one of my project called "The Aging Athlete." He has, by many accounts, declined gracefully with age. But he knows he will be slowing down more substantially, even if that occurs at age 104. Age is not something to dread. It does its thing and we adapt. As Einstein said, "Every age has its beautiful moments." Charlie French has incredible memories of his training and competitions. Could you imagine winning your age group at Ironman Hawaii in four different decades?

Charlie, an engineer by trade, likes to plan things out and develop training programs that work well over time. He took up gym workouts in his 80s and improved his endurance times markedly. Though some thrive at high intensity levels, one rarely meets high intensity older folks who are free of nagging injuries. This isn't to suggest avoiding high intensity exercise completely. Done correctly this has wondrous benefits—including causing the body to dump its own HGH (human growth hormone) into the blood stream.

This is part of the body's built-in fountain of youth. Even done once per week, this training allows for the body's own weeklong muscle "rest, repair, and toning period." Get it? Most of the beneficial work happens in the days following the intense exercise performance. A week of building, strengthening, repair, and fat burning—all for the price of only one day of oomph. How can you beat that in the busy world?

The key is to listen to your body and not your ego. The ER receives regular drop-offs of 30-year-olds who simply forgot they haven't wrestled or jumped over things for a good decade. The ER also gets its share of middle-agers and grandparents who injure themselves hoisting check-in luggage into their cars' trunks. How much time does it take to warm up and stretch? How much time does it take to heal from a strained shoulder or back?

Admittedly, time is a big issue in a person's training schedule or in their decision to do physical activities at all. And if you've signed on for interpersonal relationships, other people have to be considered. How do working couples with limited free time work things out? Close-knit couples in which only one partner decides to become a triathlete or marathon runner certainly have issues to settle. What happened to their time once used to iron out life together? Psychologists call this bonding experience *sharing quality time*. By the way, runners whose spouses don't run have 50 percent higher divorce rate.

On a family farm, our farming ancestors—who also built their own homes, barns, benches, and driveways—might have been expected to be on the clock anywhere from 10 to 15 hours per day. The difference was they were working together and they were frequently among plants, animals, wood, fabric, and leather. For the last few, think arts and crafts work done in survival and necessity mode. Working and sharing meals together, as long as the individuals are not incorrigible ogres, is part of the bonding and life-skills and life-lessons sharing time. If they were ogres, this may have prepared future workers for a normal day on the job in the factories or as wranglers on someone else's ranch.

A big difference between physical work in the family or clan and how most of us work today is that old-school farmers were maintaining their bodies, their livelihood, and their families simultaneously. We modernites spend countless years in skills training and academic courses. We study or work long days typically disconnected from physicality, and then try to piece together a family or dating life in whatever time is left over.

Some farms were atypical. In the western side of Ireland, peasants were able to grow one crop which flourished. The potato, whose cultivation was less than a full-time job, allowed families to have many children. They'd cook the potato up on fires fueled with dried turf. But, in most cases, balance was rarely a given part of life on the typical farms of livestock and fields—there was simply too much work. But there was certainly more balance in being around the land and animals than inside of drywall 22 hours per day. Where has the balance gone? Balance is a function of time. Too much time in one area—like work—means other areas of our life suffer.

Overwork away from nature leads to disconnection from the natural world and often results in heaving the rational mindset out the window. Get it—we blow fuses! You may be someone or know someone who has chosen to live in a mode that would be considered excessive or unreasonable. Are you on the edge of human physical activity, living at one of the two extremes: extreme couch potato or extreme athlete? Are you suffering a sickness or anorexia but are still exercising excessively? Do you know others who, when given the job of taking care of themselves, could be fired for incompetence? Most of us have the capacity to handle things properly, but our choices and unconscious mind drag us down.

Serial Transformers

Among the folks who are currently "couchers," there are those who could be categorized as perpetual fitness transformers, or serial transformers. Whether it's an expression of sentimentality or the best of intentions, they're always just about to get on some new kick to get moving again and drop unwanted pounds.

Some are even gym members just for the sentimental value. You've probably read the statistics on total gym membership as compared to those who actually use the facilities. Put it this way, in most gyms, if everyone who was a member used the fitness center regularly, there'd be no room to exercise. The statistics suggest only 15 percent of the members use the gym regularly.

Endless attempts at transformation—typically punctuated by tremendous weight vacillations and fitness levels—are arguably poor ways to spend considerable amounts of life's energy. What happened to common sense and taking care? Why can't humans maintain the human being? Does it make any sense that we learn to care for and drive a two-ton vehicle but never master our own personal maintenance? The 4-wheel drive truck simply has to look spotless or else. We, on the other hand, can just wear an XXL T-shirt over our rolls of fat. Never before in the history of humanity has XXL-sized apparel been so massively popular.

Where Do We Turn For Answers to Questions of Culture and Lifestyle?

Because of the capricious nature and ephemeral motivations of modern people who are up-sold by the latest news, or that "weird old tip for six-pack abs" blaring at us from the sidebar of the search engine, that question is never settled.

Busyness, multitasking, and information overload has us looking for many answers externally, which prevents us from tapping into our inner dimensions—the dimensions of reflection as well as our own innate intelligence. As we are spoon fed increasing helpings of negative practices (that we pay for on the front and back end), our capacity to reason becomes compromised and significantly reduced. All too frequently, the final steps on this path land at uncontrolled addiction. This can be categorized by an acceptance of giving up and acceptance of human unraveling, both of which are a far cry from self-mastery.

Many know how difficult it is to stop someone from eating junk food or playing digital video games, or how hard it is to get someone up off the couch to go for a walk after dinner. If you don't have people like that around, try this step. Try to stop people from one of the classic, legal addictions. Stand outside a bar at 9 in the morning with a few temperance pamphlets in hand and attempt to warn the arriving, early day drinkers not to go in.

How do you think you will do? While a few may listen to your spiel, most won't. You'll likely get sloughed off or pushed aside. They're not just addicted to alcohol; they're likely devouring the entire bar experience. Hanging out in bars—and the imbibing as well—is *their thing*.

The Coffee Crutch

Coffee at the corner café can be seen in the same light. People drink coffee not just for taste; somewhere along the line it became *their thing*. Perhaps more than any other specialty company that markets mostly takeout drinks, Starbucks has profited from this. Their business model has withstood heaps of encroachment from competition. It's not just the beans or the flavored water (which is essentially what tea and coffee are and there's nothing wrong with flavoring water). They sell the designer café experience and highly marked up food. That means whether you stop in for three hours to catch up on your laptop or tablet work or your reading, or simply to grab and run, patrons know just what the café experience is about because they have enjoyed it previously—perhaps on a daily basis.

Starbucks *excels* at selling the experience ... to the tune of some $14 billion in gross revenues in a recent year. Starbucks reportedly obtains the majority of its beans from growers who follow Coffee and Farmer Equity, C.A.F.E., Practices—a set of environmentally, socially, and economically responsible coffee buying guidelines. This all makes sense. They need sustainability to keep their bean shipments coming. Good press doesn't hurt either. If a company grows huge, let's hope they grow huge in ethics as well, not just ethics-oriented public relations campaigns. Starbucks, as most of the restaurants of the U.S., reportedly serves GMO milk. Some critics equate buying milk products like lattes at Starbucks to directly contributing funds to Monsanto—considered the biggest, baddest company by the anti-Big Ag movement.

Do you think you or those you know are addicted to coffee, the tea, the experience, or the caffeine?

Many of us don't need a caffeine wake-up jolt if we get proper sleep and exercise. Let's not forget the invigorating notion of fulfillment, and filling voids with positive pursuits. We need less fixes if we seem to like—or at least get something positive out of—our activities of daily living. Self-mastery lasts because somehow it is fulfilling. Self-mastery is the art of doing good things for your mind, body, spirit, and world that lead you on the path toward enlightenment. The path toward self-mastery is not necessarily difficult. Once one experiences the rewards of health, feeling good, and euphoria, this path becomes joy.

A close friend of mine heard my comments on coffee and filling voids. She stopped coffee and switched to organic, herbal (no caffeine) tea. After two days of withdrawal headaches and two weeks of occasional dizziness, she has been fine without coffee. Her sleep has improved and so has her morning wakeup routine. In the beginning, she played a bit of snooze roulette. Previously this meant five or six times of reaching for the snooze button during her coffee period. That evolved to fewer and fewer snooze button extensions, then disappeared entirely. Once up, she serves herself an herbal tea and then begins her exercise routine.

It's her new, accepted pattern. Do it enough and it becomes easy. Twenty-one days is all some experts say it takes. In the case of my friend, her physique, sleep patterns, and cholesterol have all improved while her wakeup and exercise routine has become easier. It's important to know some of the basic biochemistry on caffeine. The hormone cortisol is released by caffeine intake. Some call this cortisol dumping. This can cause a reaction along the same pattern of a fight or flight response. The science says this reaction can directly impact cholesterol levels in many of us. This of course can be determined via a simple blood test. Caffeine's pros and cons are easily searched on the Web. The way I read the list rounds out at more than 95 percent con, which to a so-called Spartan means it's off the list. Just say no.

About this and other questionable things we humans have been ingesting, a health conscious friend told me, "Once you get off poisons, you no longer even like the taste of them."

When I originally started a coffee counter-case for this book (and when I made the decision in my teens to never become a habitual user), I knew nothing about the history of the drink or the production methods. I went with my gut, which coffee can irritate by the way. Some innate intelligence I tapped into said, *Yes, nearly everyone's doing it. But that doesn't mean it's good for you like water.* Continuing on, I thought, *No, it's too bitter and needs too much sugar to make it taste good.*

A number of older people I knew who drank it also seemed to smoke. Perhaps this is because smoking kills your taste buds. Yuk! So, way back when, coffee never became a daily habit. Though, I did partake in coffee ice cream from time to time and dark chocolate covered espresso beans when the dessert isle at Trader Joe's tilted itself down and thrust such contents into my shopping cart.

There is a telling positive to this caffeinated concoction. Before juicing was widely practiced, how did sleepy (not yet awake; drowsy) or fatigued (worn out) people get their upper, their legal kick? Coffee can certainly provide that kick.

Even with good sleep at night, I was never one to have energy all day long in the sedentary workplace. Naps were not chic in the salaried corporate job I had in Paris back in the mid-1980s. So, after the weekly French business lunch—which was a big to-do—I habitually washed down dessert with *une noisette*, a strong, tiny cup of coffee to which one typically adds a lump *ou deux* of sugar. After those three- to five-course luncheons, how could I have functioned from 1:30 to 6 p.m. without the fix? Or perhaps it simply escorted me past the 1:30–2:30 afternoon bio-systemic need for a snooze or some mental downtime. Some cultures take the customary siesta.

By 2:30, the drowsiness had typically worn off; the *déjeuné* was getting digested and by then was providing caloric fuel. Also helpful in the late afternoon hours was that work was generally engaging me, and my departure time was on the not-too-distant horizon.

For some people, there was no other way to do it without the spark in the drink. Coffee was a compromise—a delectable one and a pleasing experience. Coffee gave them *the juice* they needed to accomplish their tasks. My cousin Henry, the former U.S. Marine I mentioned, is a fitness legend and worked for more than three decades as a federal agent. Henry has been a coffee drinker since junior high school. Just recently I found out who started him on coffee back then—my grandmother who lived right near the Catholic school and used to cook him lunch. Perhaps without seeing it in a negative way, Nell thought it culturally normal and scholastically helpful to start him on the caffeine train back in the mid-1970s. He has accomplished much professionally, athletically, spiritually, and the list goes on. Much of this could be attributed to his emotional will and physical abilities over long days fueled in part by the power of coffee.

Nutritionists and health practitioners may be shaking their heads. But if Henry makes it to 92 still achieving excellence, one could conclude that coffee worked for him. Even if he makes it to a lesser age, he will have had more than a half-century of being on task for lengthy periods, longer than many people could handle, winning elite fitness competitions along the way. By the way, he does believe in naps. Like most people in the rat race, he just couldn't take them as often as he needed them.

My other grandmother, Georgina, served my siblings and me fruit juice and tomato juice. Her daughter, my mother, never served us coffee. So, as a kid, I wound up being served juices, milk, iced tea, and healthful food. Rarely did we eat fast food. With this good start, healthful drinks were what I sought out. Like my cousin, my schedule has been that of a busy camper. Unlike my cousin, I didn't have the added commitment (and joy and worries) of raising a family. I've had lots more downtime. And because I'm not a federal agent, I've had far fewer forms to fill out and doors to batter-ram. I have yet to ask him if he's ever called out, "Freeze, dirt bag," after splintering a front door.

Cops in films notoriously drink a lot of coffee. You may recall Clint Eastwood as Dirty Harry. Here's one bit of a famous line he says to his boss who is threatening him from close proximity: "Your mouthwash ain't makin' it."

So, for the first few decades of life, my morning beverage was not coffee but orange juice and other 100 percent fruit juices. I took most them off the daily list in my early 40s when a presentation speaker asked, "We drink varying amounts of liquid per meal and in between. But do you think it's appropriate to eat six or 10 oranges in a day? Or three or four in a meal's time?" Get it; we are not designed by the historic side of nature's evolution to have that much acid and sugar hitting the system in one fell swoop. Though some anthropologists argue our predecessors—the hunter-gatherers—historically gorged on sugary foods when their fruit ripened on tree branches. Those sugar gorge sessions were seasonal, not daily or weekly throughout the year. Because of this we would be lax in calling them "gorge-ivores."

In recent times, juicing vegetables and fruits has enjoyed popularity. I do some juicing and controlled fasting and have seen good results. But my look at vegetable and fruit juicing was frappéd a bit during a presentation by Dr. David B. Agus, M.D., author of "The

End of Illness." Dr. Agus, an oncologist who treated Steve Jobs for his pancreatic cancer, mentioned the downsides of some forms of juicing: oxidizing important nutrients, rapid release of sugars, and removal of fiber.

As soon as we crush or grind up the fruits and vegetables, some of the nutrients oxidize and sugars are released. For those focused on all-around optimal health, it might be okay to enjoy the higher sugar juices on occasion, but probably not once or twice a day. For those who are impulsively less than attentive about wellness, 100 percent juice is a better way to go than junk juices and sodas. Juice made by a high-end, fiber-maintaining juicer, blender, or extractor seem the more optimal choices. Or, you can do what I have been doing. Periodically, I cycle in this drink: filtered water, a lemon, and a small amount of cinnamon. More on this later in The Sifu Slim Program for Daily Living.

Here's one of the issues with sugar. It spikes the pancreas generating first high blood sugar, then an insulin response, which lowers blood sugar. If you had your druthers, eating the fresh produce is suggested to provide more health benefits than the juice, as well as some time for masticatory enjoyment and enzymatic activity. The fiber in fruits and vegetables is essential to the digestion process and it slows down the sugar absorption. Some juice regimens add some or all of the fiber back into the juice. That's where I'd lean in the practice of juicing.

For now, remember not to bastardize all of your food. According to Dr. Agus, chew and eat fresh fruits and vegetables rather than juicing. Macrobiotics and raw fooding calls for at least 33 chews per mouthful of food. One Japanese friend's mother would encourage us to even "chew" our milk.

Once you settle on that bit of knowledge, you are jarred out of your seat of accepted health practices once again by watching a moving documentary film such as "May I Be Frank" or "Fat Sick and Nearly Dead." These programs show fellow people who are miserably unwell and eventually can't stand it anymore. Both of these *transformational* documentaries touch on death (and the miserable path toward it) as the big motivator for change. With the power in juicing and controlled, physician-monitored juice fasting, love of self, and loving support, people change their mental and physical health and regain wellness and their lives. Put these two documentaries on your list to watch.

The Soapbox Standoff— Coffee vs. 100 Percent Juice

For some of us, coffee should be consumed on the rare occasion ... perhaps when cramming for a final exam, or when you're heading south on I-95 in the winter and have to get to Florida to thaw out. Still, sleep is the miracle potion, not coffee. Don't drive tired or amped up on caffeine. Pull in to the rest area, shade your eyes with a sleeping beanie or scarf, cover yourself with a blanket or three, and snooze as much as you need.

Many have been jarred awake by the sound of another car's horn or the sounds of stones from the side of the freeway that are pelting the car's undercarriage or wheel wells. You're in a 60 mile-per-hour bullet. You awaken to find the bullet you are driving is now driving you and together you're headed toward a guardrail, a tree, or the back of a semi. Now that's scary!

Your pancreas thinks a heavy sugar dump is equally foreboding. Realizing that concentrated, fiber-free sugar is seen as a pandemic problem, how can one answer the following question? Are bottled, 100 percent juices better than coffee for us? You'll have to forgive me since I am climbing upon a soapbox to warn that for some people that's like asking, "Is it better to get punched in the gut or punched in the face?"

They're both probably better than chemicalized, sodium-rich, sugarized sodas—a punch in the teeth, a kick in the groin, a potential expensive trip to the dentist and endodontist, and an early nail in the coffin. There are healthful sodas on the market known for great tastes. But remember, it's likely that even health products use food science to sharpen taste. If you must drink soda, drink the healthful varieties. They're quite tasty—to me much tastier than the usual suspects that have sought to own part of our pocketbooks and souls.

What does one look for on the label to determine whether a variety of soda is "the healthful variety"? Unless it is explained, some readers will justify to themselves that artificially sweetened, zero calorie soda from Coke and Pepsi counts as healthful. Typically, none of this is good for you.

Don't look for the words "natural" or "healthy." They don't mean much since a company may be able to get away with using such enticing words with far too much leeway. Go to farms themselves, farm stands, farmers' markets. Also, get acquainted with the smaller, less-corporatized healthful markets that are hopefully available in your area.

Then try Trader Joe's, Whole Foods, and other more large-chain purveyors whose rows feature some proportions of healthful options. Read the labels on the glass bottles in these stores. Yes, glass bottles. Because of potential leaching, you want to use glass, not aluminum or plastic. To the avoidance list, include these banes: non-natural preservatives, chemicalized coloring, added flavors, consistency agents, bad acids, caffeine, and corn syrup. Especially steer clear of other horrible sweeteners like aspartame and sucralose.

You may be aware that some school districts across America have banned the junk sodas and caffeine drinks from their campus restaurants and vending machines. That means they're getting smarter in a few areas. At some point we'll probably see cell phone towers come down from their rooftops—too much EMF exposure. When will they start preparing real food again? Maybe this will follow when two things happen:

The government takes some of the people's money out of destinations such as war and spends it on education and food.

We get the food corporations to provide real food from organic farmers instead of the pre-prepared boxed junk that most schools are currently serving.

In my philosophy for healthful living, it's not solely about what tastes good or what *most* people do that drives the adopted or continued custom. Remember the last time your bowels erupted or were blocked up in the bathroom? Remember the last time you fell asleep in the meeting due to insufficient sleep or low blood sugar?"

I recently told a friend that I sometimes run a bit prone to melancholy and sleepiness, perhaps by nature.

His take: "Your brain is burning lots of energy. It's the most energy consuming organ in the body."

"Yeah," I answered, "I have a busy mind."

"How is your metabolism?"

"Because of my fitness program and innate high metabolism,

I normally have to consume a lot of food. The digestion process also tires me out and my caloric requirements put a nice dent in the monthly budget."

"Well," he offered, "the brain uses lots of glucose, so you may wish to try smaller meals like body builders do." This statement runs counter to my claims of being fat-adapted, being able to derive energy from the body's fat stores.

"And meditation," I suggested. "I have that on my list."

"Meditation is key. I do it with my guitar—I get into a trancelike state when I'm playing."

"Dehydration is another problem. One of its side effects is fatigue," I suggested.

"What are you going to do about that?" he asked.

"I'm going to soak my active head and busy abdomen in the Pacific. In fact I may move aboard the Sloop John B so I can jump in on the hour. Maybe catch me some kelp. Good for the thyroid. Maybe give me some zing."

Do You Ever Stop to Consider Your Internal Wellness?

What is the best energy-boost drink on the market today?

It's the power nap of course.

If that is too quick, consider the longer version, a siesta. A nap is a great provider of alertness, relaxation, readiness, and smoothness. And, yes, you can be alert and relaxed at the same time.

We have smart cars, why not smart homes and offices? Naps should be taken when we need them, daily, not just when we are sick or completely exhausted.

Needing your fix of coffee to keep awake or gain energy may be an indication your body's energy-making centers are down—your adrenals are failing. The adrenal glands found atop your kidneys produce hormones that stimulate energy and alertness. Coffee cravings and daily trips to the coffeemaker may be signs of adrenal burnout, a condition that results in fatigue. This fatigue results from conditions and activities that may include undiagnosed chronic infections, poor nutrition, improper exercise, and overwork. Such draining life patterns overtax the adrenals to the point they fail to function properly. Overstressed, they are unable to keep their hormone production in proper balance.

What are we programmed to do when we're drained during the fulfillment of our daily tasks?

We caffeinate ourselves or sugar snack, of course! Have you taken note of the proliferation of energy boost drinks over the past decade? They're just what our younger generation needs to remain spiked and plugged into the matrix. Unfortunately, high schoolers are a big market for these drinks. You know, Red Bull, Monster, and Rockstar. Annual sales of soda are down but energy drink sales have been on the rise.

It's easy to draw a parallel that links high school students and energy boosts with adrenal fatigue. If adrenal fatigue is happening among high school students, and students are allowed to self-medicate to get a boost of an upper, that's a huge problem.

I spent a lot of time studying and writing reports in high school. I also spent a lot of time doing daily physical movement, athletics, farm work, and sleeping. Fortunately, I got better at most of this over time and never used caffeine. As far as handling the demands and culture of school, it got easier with each year. That's from age four to age, well, today. I still enroll in classes. I'm just a bit choosier about classes mostly based on the assigned workload. Some classes are simply too demanding in terms of the amount of material you are required to memorize. If the workload is excessive, life quickly gets out of balance.

In our society that is based in the mentality of more is more, more work has been considered superior. That's a preposterous notion. It's also overkill. More memorization does not translate to better ability to access and retain that information. Understanding concepts, developing mental acuity, and expanding one's mind is far superior to uploading vast megabytes of data.

"You are worried about seeing him spend his early years in doing nothing. What! Is it nothing to be happy? Nothing to skip, play, and run around all day long? Never in his life will he be so busy again."
—Jean-Jacques Rousseau, from his book "Emile."
(1712 Geneva – 1778 Ermenonville, France)

Rousseau, a leading French philosopher of the enlightenment, was talking about children playing. Have you ever seen a senior citizen who is the life of the party or the wedding? When are we too old to play?

Back in high school, I had a lot of free time during the school day to get work done. In my junior year, I had over two hours of what was known as G.A.I.N. time—Going Ahead Independently. It was so useful a program they have since done away with it. My personal opinion is that society's working systems are often reworked until they don't work. A Peter Principle of policy?

I used my G.A.I.N time to complete my schoolwork, apply to colleges, talk to teachers and friends and teammates, read on my personal interests, and organize my life. Those hours were in addition to lunch. I had it made.

After class time, I was able to concentrate on sports. Then I'd get myself home for a great dinner from M.O.M. and enjoy mealtime with my parents and my sisters. After dinner, at this point in my life, I wasn't perpetually subjected to a homework pummeling, as I would later experience in college. Because of free time during the school day, most of my work was done before school ended.

At night, I often had time to read my schoolbooks, or connect with friends and family, or just spend some quiet time on hobbies. It was nice having time to take our English setter for a walk with a flashlight, look up at the stars, and say goodnight to the natural world.

If you talk to some high school kids today, even four hours after school isn't always enough to get through the workload of six classes. During my years in high school, there were semesters in which I only had four classes. Same thing for college. Was this a better way for me? You're darned tootin'! Was I less scholastically and intellectually adept than the pummeled kids today? Heck no. Fortunately, I was a focused, yet balanced student, and I wasn't over-programmed to the same degree. There were some periods of deep personal stress and peer pressure, don't get me wrong. But, I had sufficient time to deal with education and growing up.

Now, most of the schools I am familiar with—including my alma mater in New Jersey—no longer have such programs during the school day. Some offer early dismissal for jobs or junior college classes. Schools don't want kids on campus to be unsupervised. It's a liability issue and some parents and guardians are ready and willing to sue. If students are on school grounds, the administrators want these students in class where they can be watched. And, I might add, driven too hard and asked to be on task for too many hours per day.

Most of these hours are seated. Schools, as I continue to mention, are the training grounds for the sedentary world. Do you think that schools should operate this way? Do you believe that kids should just have to deal with it?

But before you think that way, try it yourself. Go sit all day in classes for two weeks with a high school student. You can be a volunteer for a special needs student or just shadow a relative. Just sitting with a student is one thing. Being responsible for the course work and taking up all of the other things that a student handles is much more demanding. Imagine taking that on with hormones raging, growth spurts, fatigue, serotonin fluctuations, and peer pressure. You may already be familiar with this challenging experience.

Stimulation and Fatigue

What is the relationship between upper drugs and human fatigue? Energy drinks contain legal stimulants, including high quantities of caffeine and sugar. Sugar is a tricky substance since it is considered a depressant that can produce stimulating effects, especially when it's ingested with artificial colorings and additives. Our cardio systems and other systems power up to rid the artificial chemicals from our bodies. That's how the junk sugar drinks fire our cylinders. After a spate of health incidents related to these drinks—including heart palpitations, high blood pressure readings, and even cardiac arrest—some countries have banned high-energy drinks.[5]

Are people smart enough to handle their use of addicting and harmful drugs? Given how addiction works, obviously not. Intelligence needs to be bolstered by self-control. This means not only that you have able brains but also that you can efficiently manage what the impulsive brain is telling you.

How smart is the department chair university professor who sneaks street-purchased oxycodone into her office when she needs a pop? How skillful and masterful are athletes who are hooked on drugs or doping?

"A man wrapped up in himself makes a very small bundle."
—Benjamin Franklin
(Boston, Mass. 1706 – Philadelphia, Penn. 1790)

To Franklin's quote I add: A man who resists working on himself and giving of his gifts is a bundle of low worth.

Sleep and Sports Drinks

These for-profit concoctions—which generate heap big profits—are pervading the shelves and soda machines of the world. Some drinks say they'll improve performance. What might your cardiac system answer to that? What happens when the effects wear off?

Consider for a moment that flashy concoctions are marketed as sport drinks, energy drinks, athletic drinks, and even sexual-performance drinks. Should a 21-year-old need such a drink to perk up before going out to dance clubs? Should kids have access to these quantities of drugs, sugar, and chemicals—distributed in a flashy, user-friendly can or bottle? No, said Denmark, Turkey, and Uruguay who made them illegal. These policy makers are not idiots. They know the profit game that is being played and how big money players can kill us or ruin our health.

What about illegal uppers? Why should people need these things? That's a huge question with endless books written on the subject. Stimulants—like cocaine and crystal meth—sometimes wind up in the hands and pockets of the users who show signs of being overstressed and under-recreated. The surveys say that plenty of people are dissatisfied and under-rested. Sleep has a great deal to do with satisfaction, and satisfaction has a lot to do with sleep. Many health experts promote early to bed, early to rise. I'm a big believer in getting restful and adequate sleep.

Sleeping, just like proper diet and exercise, is assisted when it becomes a repeatable pattern.

Here are some quick sleep tips on how to fall asleep:

1. Take a warm-water bath or shower to help your body temperature decrease, slow down your metabolic rate, and bring on tiredness.[6]

2. Have some chamomile tea. You can also stick some chamomile leaves in your pillowcase.

3. Insulate the room for quiet or use a white noise machine. A Kenmore Heppa Supreme air filter from Sears provides white noise and air filtration.

4. Darken the room with curtains or shades. Wear a sleeping beanie.

5. Avoid alcohol, sedatives, caffeine, and chemicalized drinks.

6. Develop a routine.

We know that our recent and ancient ancestors often slept in rooms and spaces with more noise and more people. Our different levels of sleep are due in part to a programming that allows us to handle the noise. Being accustomed to the stimuli can make us impervious to them. So, the listed darkness and noise aids are a modern compromise to our historical adaptations of sleeping.

An airplane ride can cause states of irritability and restlessness. I took the Greyhound ($12 in 2013) from Reno to Sacramento after having done a combination of six flights to, in, and from Europe. The flights were interspersed over an 8-week period and some of them were shorter than the Reno to Sacto bus trip.

To me, the half-full, new, quiet bus Greyhound provided was more relaxing than even an upgrade on Lufthansa.

The downsides of flying:

1. Air pressure
2. Recycled Air
3. Too crowded
4. Small seats with little legroom
5. Much less to see and discern outside.

On board the bus I remarked to a fellow passenger, "Greyhound has come a long way."

In terms of airplane rides, people, especially the aged and unwell, have to be careful to avoid the perils of stationary sitting, including deep vein thrombosis.

Here is an easy tip for making your flight more pleasurable. Take a nap ahead of time. And don't forget to get a good sleep before an early-morning flight. You have to be ready for your day. A flight can be good, bad, or ugly. There's no doubt an early-morning flight is made more enjoyable by a good night's sleep. For later flights, pre-flight naps, improve a passenger's chances to sleep on long plane rides, even the dreaded red-eye flight. Exhaustion doesn't always provide excellent sleep. It depends how your physical state affects your brain chemistry, organ chemistry, digestion, bowel schedule, and stress response. Exhaustion can lead to irritability and planes can be noisy. Relaxed fatigue is an entirely different feeling than being an edgy ball of nerves.

The methodology I use for exercise sets up all of these health markers for better functionality and overall wellness. Moving and invigorating the body early in the day allows a good chance of having it work well for the rest of the day. In part for that reason, my preference is to exercise in the early morning. For years I did jiu-jitsu once or twice per week, often at midday but sometimes in the evening. At night, I'm often sufficiently tired from the morning exercise and the long day that follows. When it happens, a daily nap is an added plus. All of this creates a pattern whereby falling asleep is rarely a problem.

Hormone imbalance is another thing that impacts sleep. Keep your vitamin D levels in good standings. And remember, it's a hormone that we call a vitamin. In the non-winter months, my program normally allows for a little bit of sun every day during the early-morning workout, more when I go hiking, play golf, or do outside chores. In the dead of winter, I have to get sun when the sun is out. Do you think it odd to walk around in Southern California in January with no shirt? Women can do this wearing a sports bra or modifying the decency laws. Popping pills is probably not the best way to get vitamin D but it's considered better than not getting it. A vitamin D deficiency can cause sniffles, irritability, fatigue, sleep problems, poor bone health, and even fractures.

Daily naps have been incredibly helpful for me and are a good way to simultaneously recharge and relax while also improving nighttime sleep. Some sleep experts say to avoid exercise in the late afternoon or evening. They may be correct for some or many individuals. See what works for you. Good sex can be a workout. Would you say no to that in the evening? Would you say no to a pre-dinner jog with your parents or kids? Would you say no to your home's needs and an energy boost that had you chopping wood at nine p.m.?

In my philosophy, exercise trumps sedentism. So, because exercise has to happen, do it daily and do it at the time during your day you have available. If this creates a sleep deficit, figure out how to adapt your program to get the required sleep. Again, don't pop pills just to get to sleep. One alcoholic contact told me that he took sleeping pills because "even bastardized sleep is better than tossing and turning for hours." For people who are living out of balance, you will have to seek your own answers for these types of questions. *La vie n'est pas une longue fleuve tranquille* — Life is not a long tranquil river.

Night Owls Gone A-hooting

Plenty of my friends and contacts are avowed night owls. Others simply stay up until 11 p.m. or later because they are plugged into the matrix. Many of these people think my early-to-rise stance unfathomable. What I do is only made possible by the early-to-bed stance, which I call "living on senior time." A regular schedule of golfing with my father, or getting to work or school all caused me to get up relatively early over the course of my youth. But I didn't begin doing much early-bird fitness—on the trails or in the park by 5 or 6 a.m.—until my mid-20s when I moved to Sacramento. This is a town so hot on a summer's day that journalist Mark Twain is alleged to have said, "The sin level goes down in Sacramento in the summer as it gets so hot even Satan leaves town."

In the river city that has long been California's capital, early morning exercise was usually bearable, even in July and August where daily temperatures can climb to the low 100s. No one knows better about the unbearable heat than a guy who worked weekend community events, doing hip-hop dancing dressed in a huge, foam outfit. In my late 20s and early 30s, I had the esteemed honor of serving up the footwork and stem stylistics as The Big Tomato mascot. The City of Sacramento's nickname has long been The Big Tomato, a play on the nearby endless fields of tomatoes.

"Early-bird fitness, no way, I'm a night person," say countless people these days. "But are you really?" reply the experts. Sleep experts believe that a small percentage of night owls hold that trait by way of genetics. This is to say their energy—based on circadian rhythms—is programmed to keep them up later or even into the wee hours. And many of these owls say they get their best productivity and alertness at these hours and would of course resent being lumped in with those "whack jobs" whose neighbors see that their TV sets are on all night and their rooms are closed and dark during the day.

Bored Games, Creative Juices and Responsibilities

Some sleepologists put the night owls by genetics at about 15 percent of the population. Besides that group, there are of course others who merely adopt the night-owl lifestyle. These people are up late based on a variety of purposes including personal preference, work, habit, dissatisfaction, rebellion, or addiction.

A neighbor once admitted to me his late nights were due to

Domino's. No, he wasn't a lover of board games. Pizza, he confided, was driving him to be up until the time he felt he could binge. He said the pizza and soda were satisfying to his system. After the pizza, he could sleep. Satisfaction was both satiating and sleep inducing. Examined through a wellness microscope, the pizza binge kept him up at night.

Another person I know is a videographer. He films during the day, then crashes, then edits in the wee hours—a time he says his creative juices are flowing. There are others who take on the responsibilities of keeping things running. Some work the late shifts or graveyard shifts to keep the pumps pumping and the streets safe. Someone has to staff the hospitals, convenience stores, and 24-hour restaurants. If you work as a truck driver, your best driving hours are when fewer people are on the roads. And you have to stay alert for your entire drive time.

No matter the good intentions of those who have chosen or are forced to be awake in those hours, being up late at night has its downsides. Disrupting evolution's circadian rhythms is one. Then there's the potential dark side. Late night living can increase one's proclivities to using unhealthful products and binging as well as endlessly using digital devices. I met one night security guard who popped caffeine pills and drank Red Bull to stay awake. He told me that upper taking was rampant in his job. This isn't to throw everyone under the late-late bus, but to remind us of human tendencies so we can stave off potential pitfalls such as bad habits and addictions.

A former school principal I met moonlights from his semi-retirement as a beer tender. He told me, "I can't mix drinks, so I serve beer and clean up the bar. The tips are actually pretty good."

After sharing some thoughts with him on a variety of subjects, including Western medicine, I asked him about the late-night crowd. "You're gonna love this," he started. "We have a crew of female nurses who come in after their graveyard shift. They're in our place in the morning after they punch out."

"You're not talking coffee?" I asked.

"Nope, hard stuff, mixed drinks. Then they drive home. It's not pretty."

Late at night is a time when no one is watching. The darkness of night can obscure the realness of following best practices. Late at night leans rebellious by its very nature. Then there's attitude. Unhappy people tend to rebel more than folks who are happy and fulfilled. Plenty of folks who are battling depression or are stuck in the realm of melancholy have told me they wish they could break out of staying up late at night. One friend from Spain told me, "I go to sleep at 2 or 3 in the morning, after I'm done flipping through the remote for hours ... I eventually wake up at 10 a.m. But, if no one calls me, I sometimes sleep in till 1 p.m. At age 25, I feel like I'm wasting a lot of precious time. I need a way out of this."

According to Sarah Novak in Discovery Fit & Health, "A number of factors seem to bring the night owl down. For example, they often still have to wake up early in the morning to go to work. So much of the time they're awake, they wish they were sleeping. In other words, their life is not in line with their sleep schedule."[7] Having fought this so many times, it's easy to recall the dread. Much negativity and self-loathing was provided by missing out on the morning in my youth. "I could have been a contender ..."

Most of us have suffered this and will probably suffer this again. Life's responsibilities—or a neighbor's noise—can cause us to miss some winks. Isn't insufficient sleep a royal drag? But, since it does seem to reoccur, we adapt. That's part of why caring parents are so impressive. They do things, as one dad describes, "That are humanly impossible." They worry about their kids, lose sleep, and then respond late at night when their kids are sick or distraught.

When you miss the requisite sleep, your morning may be lackluster and your afternoon at work or school can seem like it will never end. Everything can suffer. Our cells know it, our psyches know it, even our dog knows it. The morning walk around the neighborhood is cut short and our other morning plans are put off or trimmed. It's a royal downer.

Recently, a savvy friend gave me a pep talk on this. I told him, "So many people are telling me that their schedule is just too packed. What's the answer?"

"The busier we get, the more efficient we become," he offered. "If somebody from the outside did a time-management study on you and kept an accurate journal, they would see that how you used your day is highly productive, that you were multitasking." When you are on vacation or retired, he related, "It's customary that you take a lot longer to do things ... which is okay and healthy. But take it from me, there is satisfaction in efficiency. You can get a lot of joy from it. It's not about deadlines from someone else. But the deadlines you create for yourself can give you a lot of satisfaction."

Conclusion: It's good to be efficient in our routines. It's good to get things done. The feeling of accomplishment is not just ego food; it's undoubtedly part of doing our job as a productive participant in the human race.

Addiction Blues that Can Be Rocked Out

Most of us have dealt with addiction to one thing or another—TV, alcohol, work, sex, shopping, gambling, chocolate, candy, beauty appointments, or running excessively. As far as substance abuse, it's been so common that many of us have read on the subject and attended meetings on it, whether to deal with a loved one's addiction or our own. It's highly possible, but certainly not shameful, that you've shaken hands with people at church or at work who have been users of a highly addictive drug—like crystal meth—without you even knowing about it. Though, crystal meth's side effects are normally difficult to conceal. Manufactured stimulants and illegally distributed, addicting substances run rampant in today's denatured and weary society.

I met a young, fit fellow named Matt at the beginning of a beach workout a few years ago. At the age of 22, he told me his life seemed destined for early demise. After years of drug addiction and life on the edge, Matt found a program at the Rescue Mission that helped him replace addiction with positive steps. "I was put in jail and now I'm in a program. I've been strung out on heroin for the past three to four years. And now I'm in the best shape of my life because I've sobered up. It was a good thing I was put in jail because that totally woke me up."

What I got from Matt is that he wanted meaning and wanted to feel good. He said, "Before, I would have never thought that working out would be as fun as it is." He had taken out a gym membership and was running the football stadium stairs at the junior college in Santa Barbara. And while in the program, he had a job at the Rescue Mission. As Matt explained, "Right now, you run every day, you do weight training, and you see results. If you want to get in shape, just do it. It gets fun. At some point, you'll see results and you'll want more."

As has already been put forth, my stance is that humans have an innate drive (and need) to seek euphoria. We can make the choice to get it in positive ways if we learn how. If you've never had it naturally, you may want to start with basic happiness. Though this seems unfathomable, there are some who have never experienced euphoria naturally. If this is you, go out and get a massage. There again is a possible holdback since some people don't like to be touched.

If the idea of a massage doesn't appeal to you, then set your intention to find out why. To do so may bring you a better understanding of yourself. If you do wind up finding a way to receive and even give a proper massage, both may provide great, natural joy and release. Psychologists have concluded the lack of touch retards development in infants and children. Lack of touch can lead to negative interpersonal and biochemical outcomes—including disagreements and ill feelings. The brain chemistry shows that touch stimulates activity in the frontal cortex and also causes the pituitary gland to release oxytocin, known as the love hormone. We in America have experienced a growing trend of less touch, and more brain illness and stress. It's also becoming more common for some families and friends to use more touch in greetings.

Physical people tend to get physical. I remember that when I was practicing karate kicks, I'd sometimes greet people with a high kick that I held in the air at head height. It was not a kick to touch them, but one of a holding posture. It sounds nuts but it was quite natural to me and it was a bonding move of endearment and comfort. If you hold your foot up high, you are at your opponent's mercy. Once, a friend grabbed my foot and tried to throw me back. Luckily, I was able to hold on to him. Years later, I learned that Bruce Lee performed the high controlled kick when he greeted his contacts.

Some scientists think humans are programmed for laziness. Even if we are, remember how much more fun it is to be "lazy" after physical activity. If nothing physical is accomplished during the day, it's quite natural to feel lousy in body, mind, and spirit. A significant part of a being human is being physical. Negating or denying this sets us up for undoing the nature of being human.

Getting in touch with the various parts of our natural selves works wonders and typically starts showing benefits in the first day. Now, a few months into his program, Matt had gone from the weight he entered jail—140 pounds due to severely unhealthful practices—to his current fit and muscular weight of 173. "Working out is a lifestyle," Matt said. "You have your whole life to build from. I just remember feeling so good after working out." His part-time job was working with the food service of the Rescue Mission, helping to nourish others in recovery as well as nurturing himself. What a way to get a charge out of life.

What Is the Most Common Stimulant of Recent Times?

Caffeine. Remember, sugar is *not* considered a stimulant. It's a depressant.

Dr. Donald Liebell, D.C., who works in complementary and alternative medicine (and has a strong Web presence with a great deal of helpful information) was one of the first readers of Sedentary Nation. He was kind to respond to my questions about coffee.

"I cringe at people using it to wake up," wrote Dr. Liebell from his office in Virginia Beach. "Though, I'm not anti-coffee from the perspective of enjoying a hot drink, preferably organic coffee. The major causes of adrenal burnout are chronic infections, which go undetected, and even when found, ineffectively treated."

What does Dr. Liebell suggest instead of coffee to boost energy?

"I'm a fan of fresh vegetable juicing rather than devitalized vitamin supplements. People certainly hurt themselves with artificial energy in the same way they can hurt themselves with artificial health by covering symptoms with pharmaceutical drugs."

We know sugary additives and chocolate toppings can spike our pancreas, central nervous system, and personality. Caffeine may get us through long meetings and taxing commutes, but at what cost?

What Works?

In the end, even better if you find it in the beginning, you will have to embrace a lifestyle that works for you and those dear to you.

Without wellness in our lives, we assemble at medical clinics when we break down. *Perhaps they have a pill or injection to mitigate the venom building up in our veins.* Toxicity pervades our surroundings. It's everywhere: in our soil, water, air, carpets, and cells. Only one person I knew back in third grade claimed to have, or showed the signs of, asthma. Today it's widespread and often considered related to our toxic environments, poor dietary customs, and sadly inadequate physical fitness. Toxicity is even found in our social lives. Many of us are involved in toxic relationships that produce venomous emails and voice and text messages that raise ire. What can be done about all this toxicity? How do we break the pattern?

This book hammers home the idea of natural living. The idea here is not to do one or two things to overcome your woes, but to simply live in a more historically natural way. Fitness pioneer Jack LaLanne (1914–2011) used humor to answer part of this question: "If man made it, don't eat it." I don't know if he spent much time texting in his last few years of living. My guess would be that he didn't.

What are some of the main things we can do to help relieve stress?

Physical activity, recreation, relaxation techniques, and social bonding will all work. Time has to be set aside to handle such activities. If you plan out the day properly, you can carve out time for a moment of de-stressing. If you don't plan it out, where are you at the end of the day? Stressed and feeling guilty that everyone and everything got taken care of but you!

An ostensibly congenital problem of modern Homo sapiens is that we are too often reactors instead of planners. We go to group therapy when we're already unable to cope with anxiety. Do we deny that life is stressful and deny that things such as letting off steam and bonding need to happen daily? This short-term focus is observable in how we handle the lesser issues that come up. We often sweat the little stuff, and we often take ourselves too seriously. Historically speaking, if we are out of sync, why not change course? We can dance like cave people and do some actual sweating. If an idle mind is the devil's workplace, whose is the heavy heart? The cardiac surgeon's of course. From there, the undertaker is often right around the corner followed by saddened family and friends.

An Argument to Stand By

Many stuck in sedentary pursuits are inactive, trapped inside a building most of the time, and now require meds. This is the number one problem of our current health crisis: We're a medication nation and a consultation nation (as in therapy for problems), not a movement nation. Yes, diet is important. That's for certain. But food is enjoyable and necessary fuel for physical and mental activity, not a surfeit of fuel you cram inside a barely puttering motor of a tethered barge. Natural living models completely miss the majesty of the panoramic view if they excessively focus on the act of eating organically and neglect physical culture. The history of food is inseparable from the history of movement.

The Original Action Step

The message to embrace comes from what previous generations of humans—the hunter-gatherers and then the farmer-ranchers—did every morning. They got up and moved their bodies to acquire food to feed their hungry selves and families. Movement meant food.

That makes sense, doesn't it?

Now go back to the oldest bones, those of the earliest upright walkers, and you'll discover a date many suggest to be more than 6 million years ago. The big story of modern wellness is that upright walkers moved, every day, for millions of years—and then, as if a slumber dust had been sprinkled on their descendants, modern people somehow stopped moving, all in a half-century. This was the later part of the 20th century.

Does that make any sense?

Does lumbering around the house or jobsite generate health and wellness? Not unless our house has fifteen floors and no elevator (and we don't abuse our bodies), not unless we work on the loading docks (and don't abuse our bodies). For moneymakers in sedentary jobs, a shuffle or amble to the refrigerator leads to filling the stomach. Nothing to do with speed afoot or arm strength. This establishes the disconnection from how for millions of years, serious movement was directly related to food. Do you remember seeing the image of a mule or horse chasing a dangling carrot held out in front of the pulling animal on a pole? This is how the "Little Rascals" (aka "Our Gang" comedy) got their rickety wagon pulled around.

What happened to the fulfilling nature of physical movement that came with the search for food? Can it be found in the gym?

These days, young people (including the crumb crunchers and their older siblings) are rarely taken to where food comes from unless you speak of the supermarket. There along the endless rows of boxes and cartons, excited youngsters invariably reach for what they crave: sugar-filled food. If they don't get their way, if a pull from mom or dad ushers them away, neighboring shoppers might very well be treated to an expressive movement form known as a tantrum. Now that's a far cry from softly stalking game in the woods or merrily gathering eggs in the chicken coop, or pulling vegetables from a garden.

The Digital Divide

Do the young folks nearest to you know much about old-school farms or the hunting and gathering of native people? It's more likely you'll come across those who excel at finding the fridge, the couch, and digital entertainment. Is such a lifestyle the most pervasive revulsion of our times? Is this a peek into the potential of the overpopulated world's devolution (some call this dysevolution), or is it simply a new branch of our space-efficient evolution?

Nielsen's ratings show that the average American household in the new millennium boasts 2.93 television sets, up from 1.75 in 1975. Does it startle you when you read: "Since at least 2005, there have been more TVs per household on average than people per household"? [8] Is this devolution growing in strength or, instead, nearing its climactic fall? Big things to consider as you turn the pages.

Readers may be relieved to hear that there won't be an overuse of the word *lazy*. Over-programmed, yes; subject to addiction, yes; but not a continued harping on laziness. Sedentary living and fitness avoidance run deep, and they appear to present entirely different rationale as compared to not taking out the trash or cleaning the home.

Devoid of quiet, peaceful, communal downtime—together with fitting in so many responsibilities we seem forced to do on our own (in many cases, with no more villages or families joining together to handle daily tasks)—many of us are overwhelmed in our average day. Since most jobs are not physical, many of us are inactive balls of atrophy topped by restless minds. Many are also loners and live lives devoid of meaningful social interaction. Socializing has been singled out as the major commonality among societies steeped in centenarians: Okinawa; Sardinia; Nicoya, Costa Rica; and Loma Linda, California. [9]

Living far from family (or in the midst of family dysfunction) and only socializing through digital media seems to cause our dipsticks of meaning to run dry. Can money fill the void? Most of us would take money over poverty, but according to some singers from Liverpool, money can't buy us love.

The couch, chair, and bed are seen as places to rest our royal hindquarters and mind from some of the busyness. Those comforts are always there for us ... beckoning. And because we spend too many hours sitting and lying around, we suffer the aches and pains of dysfunction that has us popping pills, or when that provides no more relief or winds up messing up our internal body systems, doing rehabilitative therapy. Runner's World writer Selene Yeager says, "Sitting Is the New Smoking." She aptly opens her article: "There's no running away from it: The more you sit, the poorer your health and the earlier you may die, no matter how fit you are."[10]

And if sitting around is not bad enough, long periods of standing have been linked to a litany of ailments, including increased chance of stroke.* If you are stuck in a life of sitting in front of computer and T.V. screens, do you want to pull away? The prudent seeker of balance will take periodic breaks from the perpetual digital onslaught and endless multitasking? Imagine going for a walk sans your smartphone. Or are the picket fence and front porch of the American Dream only available via smartphones?

Go Out and Get Some Outdoor Living

Regardless of our employment situation, can't we step away from drywall and concrete and spend some time, both moving and resting, under trees, in parks and fields, and along trails? Wise old Ben Franklin, a proponent of mental and physical recreation, himself a former weightlifter, would say "Hear, hear!" to that.

If exertive and sustained movement leads to invigoration, a sexier bod, and a natural high, why has modern living ushered in

---

* Sources claim carotid atherosclerosis, plaques, and other disruptive substances accumulating in the carotid artery, increase our chance of stroke and other harmful conditions and are exacerbated by long periods of standing.

endless periods of sedentary indoor and in-car living? Is a remote control or lead foot synonymous with the ultimate of human experiences?

For humans, the indoors has its own vital relation to wellness, most notably utilized for rest, temperature control, food storage, and shelter. The indoors' association with the history of physicality is easily evidenced in such activities as dancing in a hall, breaking up wood for a cave's fire, and leather hide softening in an igloo.

But today, inside living is excessively and recurrently filled with phony worship of passing imagery. To assess the pervasiveness of visual entertainment, ask a telling question: Do you yourself want to play, or do you want to watch other people play?

Which is more invigorating? Your eyes glued to TV stars dancing and athletes playing? Or you on your own fields, trails, dance floors, yoga mats, and sports courts doing your own thing? Which provides elation with no need for chips, dip, salsa, or beer? Listen to the wise mothers who have urged for centuries, "Go out and play!" A few new millennium parents urged me to share this: Kids aren't safe like they were in yesteryear. Of course prudence is always advised.

When I asked my father, born in 1930, about the question of movement and overweight kids, here's the email I got back: "Far as I know from grammar school on there were always a few fat kids in the class. Of course we walked to school and always had gym class and had after-school sports or play in the street. Not a sedentary life at all."

If we follow our mother's advice and actually resume the kind of movement and recreation we often had as a child, what are the documented benefits for us today?

"If there's a fountain of youth," said Toni Yancey, M.D., "it is probably physical activity." Yancey, a former college basketball player, was a professor in the health services department of UCLA. She also created a program called Instant Recess (also the title of her book on wellness and movement whose subtitle is "Building a Fit Nation 10 Minutes at a Time"). Her program sets up the opportunity for everyone, especially workers in any field, to take periodic movement and stretch breaks—and have a blast doing it. While I was in contact with her for my next book, "The Aging Athlete," she passed away in her 50s. This goes to show that we all can be taken at any time.

Research on exercise has shown specific benefits to every organ system in the body—heart, brain, lungs, and even sexual organs.

According to Dr. Yancey: "We just aren't really structured to be sitting for such long periods of time, and when we do that, our body just kind of goes into shutdown."

What are some of the benefits of daily exercise?

1. Lower stress and blood pressure
2. Improved cardiovascular and lymphatic health
3. Improved posture and stronger supportive structure
4. Improved digestion and elimination
5. Improved levels of cholesterol and triglycerides
6. Improved bone density and bone health
7. Reduced age-related disease risk
8. Reduced risk of diabetes and certain types of cancer
9. Looking good and feeling even better

But Is Daily Exercise and Physical Activity Enough?

96

Not if you are sitting or standing all day.

A study found prolonged sitting is a link to a greater risk of kidney disease and death. In this same study, researcher Emma Wilmot, M.D. points out the average adult spends between 50 and 70 percent of their day sitting down. What can be done then to prevent this scenario from unfolding? Thomas Yates, M.D., who led the study, tentatively recommends standing for two minutes for every 20 minutes you're sitting down and even standing during TV commercials when that's possible. More realistically, any break from sitting can be beneficial, even if it's just to stand for a few seconds.

Some researchers whose names were mentioned in a Wall Street Journal article suggest 30 minutes of exercise per day to help "beat heart attacks." Columnist Ron Winslow suggests as far as duration that even 10 minutes per day can help. "While the 30-minute target is associated with a 70 percent reduction in heart-attack risk over a year, Mayo researchers analyzed the data and noticed that a brisk 10-minute walk a day results in a nearly 50 percent reduction compared with people who get hardly any exercise."[11]

A response to these findings: Teach people these physical movement practices when they are young. Indoctrinate them just as we do with nearly everything else. In fact, do this particular teaching even better than the other sources of indoctrination. We know we have to eat, or our bodies shut down. The same thing goes for physical activity.

Don't be permanently sedentary. Get up and move. Health experts tell us to get up and move about and stretch during long airplane flights because they know the harm that sitting causes. (In 2014, this practice was banned on many flights "due to security measures.") Sitting all day presents the same problem. Lengthy standing presents other problems.

One of the situations where sitting can actually be beneficial to your health and wellbeing is when you practice *conscious breathing.* Although this can be done standing or lying down, sitting is probably the easiest way of quickly adapting it to your regular routine.

This deep breathing discipline has a long record of improving wellness in Chinese and now Western medicine. At its most basic, it relieves stress and tension. Similar to sustained exercise, conscious breathing strengthens the immune system and enhances the lymphatic system, part of the body's circulatory system that carries lymph fluids toward the heart. This is essential for healing and good health—and staying alive. Moreover, this type of breathing helps modify and calm the messages the vagus nerve sends from the gut to your brain. Since the vagus nerve has such a profound effect throughout our parasympathetic nervous system, including heart rhythm, this alone merits our full attention.

Wellness consultant Dr. David Beamer has adopted conscious breathing at its most complete level and describes the proper technique this way:

1. Relax the lower muscles of your abdomen.
2. Breath in through *your nose,* filling the lower portion of the lungs first. This will result in your *abdomen expanding* out as your diaphragm drops down and compresses your internal organs.
3. Then allow the upper lobes of the lungs to fill as you draw the air (again only through your nose) *up into your chest* cavity.
4. Hold for a couple of seconds (to avoid any lightheadedness), then *exhale slowly through your mouth.*

5. Repeat and gradually deepen and slow the breath.[12]

Try to work up to *at least 21* of these breaths back to back and combine them with five other single *remembering breaths* throughout the day—so named because they remind your body of the major benefits the conscious breathing has already effected.

A friend who has been seeing the benefits of this for years tells those who whine they don't have time for that: "Okay, why not just do it on the days you breathe?"

Rather than our commonplace shallow breathing, this is how we should breathe as often as possible. By the way, this friend does 35 of the conscious breaths four or sometimes five times a day and swears by the health benefits.

Important Tip on Exercises to Engage the Body

Do standing knee ups, jumping jacks, trunk twists, yoga and Pilates stretches, low-impact karate kicks, balanced punches from the horse stance, shadow boxing … anything that gets your body moving. People talk about walking. Of course it has positive benefits, including clearing the mind, getting the blood flowing, and resetting the joints. But we often do it on flat surfaces. Walking up hills and stairs should be mixed in with your flat walking.

To pump more exhilaration into your walking, try some of these techniques:

1. Go fast up inclines.
2. Move your arms in a coordinated manner. Think Fred Astaire mixed with cross-country skier, not a lunatic on leave.
3. Carry hand weights and do exercises with them as you walk.
4. Hold two folded tube socks in each hand. (Folded once and

then twisted twice works for my medium-large hand size.) Firmly and smoothly squeeze from pinkie to thumb. This strengthens hands and arms and helps prevent carpal tunnel and some forms of arthritis.

5. Periodic shadow boxing, controlled lunges, or jumping jacks exert even more physical effort and produce more muscle contractions as well as cardiovascular and biochemical benefits. There's also nothing wrong with throwing in some incline pull-ups on a horizontal bar or tree branch and some incline push-ups on a wall or park bench.

See how I coach? Get a walker walking with more huffing, and then get them puffing with some actual exercises. The more you use your muscles, the more efficient they become. I've had women who say they don't want to get bigger muscles from exercising. I've received calls from them only a few weeks into my program. Some say things like, "I'm getting ripped. I can pick up my children, and I'm wrestling with my husband." One told me, "My husband wants into the program. He wants to flex in the mirror with me ... I can't believe I'm doing that, but I am."

Imagine a house off the electrical grid. The wife and the husband are not happy with something that has come up between them. You know, something that's a big deal in the moment but is all but forgotten by morning. The wife tells the husband, "We're out of power, dear. Could you ...?"

The husband climbs aboard the stationary bike and begins to pedal. He generates the power the wife needs for her project. He pedals; she handles her project. Accomplishment. How much fighting and disagreeing can one do at full pedal on a stationary bike?

For the deskbound, Arizona State's Robert Ott says, "It's important to get up periodically. Taking a 15-minute break every two hours away from the computer to do a different task is a good way to vary activity."[13] Picture how architects work either standing or sitting on stools. The drafting table set-up allows for easy "stepping off" into the walking, weight-bearing realm. That's the recipe for the office potato who wants a slight sprinkle of healthful seasoning.

Some people have success using a round physio ball for desk sitting, though reports have come out stating that these balls have caused harm in numbers of people. Answer this question in your own way with common sense: Is what you are doing working for you? If it is, your body and mind will know it. If you are slouching on a physio ball, it's not the right seat for you.

This is what I, an avowed laptop potato, use. It takes the sedentary person, me, injects some molecular movement, and attempts to fool their body into thinking it's not so sedentary. Here's a bit of the actual recipe:

Do some invigorating movements (like those I mentioned previously) on the hour. As I sit here writing this, I'm reminded not just to stretch my hand to reach for a phone call that just came in. I attach my boom mike earpiece and begin doing some squats and stretches during the conversation. And do an hour of physical activity before or after work every day. Then stretch before going to sleep. Remember what Thomas Jefferson said: "health is worth more than learning."

"But the deadlines, Sifu. We're so busy!"

Okay, who isn't busy? Jack LaLanne earned the sobriquet "the godfather of fitness." Bruce Lee is the most famous martial artist of the modern era. Both Jack and Bruce had busy schedules, but they found time to exercise. Wasn't one of your great-great-grandmothers a tad busy with her umpteen young'uns on the farm? Somehow we have to do it. We have to become superhuman not just with our emails, spreadsheets, and technical skills, but we have to become adept movers of our masses.

Health is the pursuit and practice concealed behind the ever-present obstacle called performance, aka busyness. We can tune in and log in, but since serious eyes are upon us, we have to get our jobs done and our chores completed. When we do decide to do some physical movements, some part of our conscious keeps reminding us, by golly *we can't be too playful in our movements. That would be unprofessional.*

What should we do, deny ourselves physical release and simply blend ibuprofens into our smoothies? Would overloading and possibly damaging the liver be more professional?

Worn Out Like a Tire By the End of the Day ...

Can we find relief from all of this sedentary malarkey by fueling up on good offerings and by doing some huffing and puffing exercises? Or might we opt for smooth yoga-type positions that connect us with our inner selves and truth? Some people wonder if it's okay to just be active.

One technician who works in corporate ergonomics—the science of fitting machines and apparatuses (like chairs, desks, and computer screens) to human bodies—told me with a frustrated grin, "You're talking to a population of disconnected, dissatisfied people. They don't know movement the way people did a few decades ago. Today, so many people regard exercise as *offensive*."

"That's fine," I countered. "They don't have to exercise; they can recreate."

"Sure," he agreed, "that's the ticket. But there are plenty of ex jocks who don't get it. My brother was better in sports than I was. But now he's a whale and has had two bypasses and looks horrible. He calls me the jock since I still do fitness and recreation. He sits inside his home and flips channels. That's his retirement. Pretty pathetic I'd say."

"That occurrence is the subject of my book 'The Aging Athlete.'" This 62-year-old fit man had just opened the door for how my second book relates to my first book. "It's about the ten percent of ex jocks who still regularly maintain fitness which is a driver for wellness. The other ninety percent don't and many are suffering things like your brother."

Another busy person I know said this about daily fitness: "Coming home at the end of my day wired, tired, and fried makes the notion of physical movement the furthest thing from my mind." This reaction is another reason to do it first thing in the morning. Walking at lunchtime is great but it's not enough. You have to work your entire body.

An additional reader shared an opposing remark to the comment "… physical movement the furthest thing from my mind": "That's not entirely true," said the reader. "We think about it, but we don't do it. I can't tell you why. I know that if I do it, I'll feel better, but most of the time I just don't do it. If you can figure that out, I'd be your best student."

Keep reading because I've done the figuring.

The Fixed vs. Flexible Mindset

Watching countless people relapse back, away from wellness, we can draw some conclusions about how our minds work. Mindsets are either fixed or flexible. If you are negligent in your wellness and are so *fixed*, so beholden to your patterns, that you cannot seem to adopt a new mindset, then your path to wellness will be quite a challenge and will require lots of loving support, including self-love and acceptance of improvement.

Those of you who have been lax in your wellness choices but are *flexible*—and are ready, willing, and able to move into and accept the new you—will have a much easier transition. The odds still don't guarantee wellness success, but if you create a new paradigm and keep the momentum, you will have a good chance at succeeding.

Whether your particular mindset is fixed or flexible, start moving anyway. Your body can lead the mind when the mind is saying no. Listen to your body. Learn about it. Embrace it at least as much as you cherish and care for your favorite objects. In one respect, it's as though I start all over every day—in my case, the mindset has to be re-created with the first step. This is just like a trolley car driver who pulls out of the station on Tuesday morning. It's a whole new day.

Because it's a matter of faith, self-love, respect, and doing the right thing, I simply have to keep my daily fitness habit going no matter what. That means I do it no matter what's pulling on my mind and filling my schedule. I do the movement program because I know the wonders this creates. I prioritize it, making sure it is the first thing on the agenda. That way I know it will get done and my hip won't malfunction while getting out of my seat ... or lock up when climbing over the side of the bathtub.

Physical movement will change parts of your chemistry and anatomy and decrease your stress level starting with your first steps. But as far as adopting a daily practice of movement and making it a daily priority you can't live and thrive without, realize that you have to accept the big mystery of wellness as truth: You feel better and look better because you have gotten out of your home (away from your stuff) and moved your body.

This is the essential concept, and you won't "get it" until you get it. When you do get it, you will, by then, arrive at a destination called a whole new you. A bit of the movement program can be done indoors. But if we are denatured, getting *natured* means stepping outside and being around things that spring forth from the earth and the skies. We are supposed to be in nature so get in nature—or at least outdoors—as much as possible.

Good fortune and long-term wellness rationality has provided me the mindset required to put this together. I spend the time necessary to "get it" every day. Without it, I'd be unbearable, in pain, disabled, or in the hereafter. By doing my maintenance movement program, I get an incredible gift: I get to be a brand spankin' new me every morning. The body and mind characteristically respond by operating on all cylinders. Then there are the other identifiable benefits including youthfulness, de-stressing, and the upbeat attitude. This is all welcome news. The body stays streamlined, flexible, and fit. I personally am grateful for this program! If you are not doing this, please contact me for coaching. Perhaps I can help.

If you are open to this type of thinking, there's a story I'd like to share with you. It's the tale of the history of physical movement that led us to sedentism. And then, I'll offer a modern answer to our lack of movement. It's the story of a working mindset that combines the passion and practice of Jack LaLanne and Bruce Lee … and lots of uncontrollable laughter, aka silliness.

Easy Takeaways

1. Look for a lifestyle and food that are not denatured.

2. Quiet downtime is important. The hunter-gatherers tended to enjoy this more than we.

3. Get outside frequently and in all seasons. We are diurnal creatures: historically awake in daytime and asleep at night; outside during the day, inside at night.

4. Coaches are always important. They help you with self-mastery. Are you coachable?

5. The way most people handle their coffee crutch is not good, and neither is the way much of it is produced. As with nearly everything done on economies of huge scale, corners are frequently cut. Look up its growing and distribution and you may get de-beaned.

6. We lethargic humans generally do the same set of things every day. We need sleep (including naps), more downtime, and wellness, not mass-produced uppers.

7. Get your fix of euphoria the natural way—move your body and your mind will follow. At some point the mind, body, and spirit will connect, and then you will know what the Zen workout is all about. It can lead to a Zen lifestyle.

8. Stay away from digital overload. It's okay to check emails, balance accounts, and read the news. It's not okay to live on

the Net or drive while texting. Addiction needs to be treated as addiction, not sloughed off.

9. Do you want to play? Or do you prefer to sit (and drink and eat) while you watch others play, aka TV sports and "Dancing with the Stars"?

10. Physical activity is the fountain of youth. And per Jack LaLanne and many others who were actively having sex into their advanced years, it's good for the sex drive.

11. Prolonged sitting and standing are detriments. Change positions frequently. If sitting, periodically change seats/chairs, and then work a bit while standing. Rotate through sitting and standing positions, and do stretch breaks and walk breaks on the hour or every two hours. For the static anatomy, the more movement the merrier.

Chapter 3

Readers' Comments and the Timeline of Decreasing Physical Movement

Here's where I try the old sales pitch—"others are doing it with successful results, so can you."

Readers' comments on the Sifu Slim message and on the book, Sedentary Nation:

"Your points are excellent and your style and flow are genuine. Your message comes across just like you'd be talking with someone in person. I don't think it's too hard-hitting—just makes the reader more aware, and it gave me many things to think about."

—Rosemarie R., busy mother and part-time employee

"A big relief came over me while reading your book. You're not just telling people to exercise, you talk about living a balanced life including

taking siestas and enjoying downtime away from digital gadgets and invasive noise. That has helped me immensely."

—Taylor Reaume, owner of Search Engine Pros, who admits, "Nearly my entire work life is spent online."

"I took two laps around Bundt Park this morning with my dog thinking: movement ... activity ... clear the head ... life is good ... burning calories ... getting fresh air ... I'm so glad I quit that unbearable job and am getting into the wellness groove. I am no longer a member of the Sedentary Nation."

—Valerie, a busy mom from Clinton, N.J.

As a rational human being, I am not suggesting everyone quit their jobs, especially in economically challenging times—but when aren't times so? Don't quit ... unless it's the best option. In this case, Valerie's 25-plus-year sedentary job was becoming increasingly unhealthful. Instead of treating a seasoned and dedicated employee with some reverence and gratitude, the corporation decided to pile on more work (after letting go of some other employees), expecting more and more, faster and faster, and continuously intruding on already limited family time during her nights and weekends. Here's the situation she described to me:

Daily communications arrived fast and furious in multiple formats, demanding immediate attention. Phones, faxes, and alarms rang, and instant-messaging bars flashed across the computer screen. Cables, plugs, and equipment engulfed the workspace, and employees were physically tethered to their desks by headsets. I could hardly think straight anymore. I often sat in a fixed position without getting up for seven to eight hours at a stretch, just to keep up with the constant onslaught and demands. I found it increasingly difficult to manage the stress and anxiety levels that were mounting. Joy was being zapped out of my life. I often felt lethargic and drained within the first few hours of my workday, but I knew I had to keep going anyway. On and on I went, day after day, year after year, in a state of emotional and physical disrepair.

Valerie's mind and body were being overwhelmed until she finally felt forced to resign. Getting her health back and spending more quality time with her 12-year-old daughter, her husband, and the rest of her family who lived in the area, has put this woman in her 50s back on track. She told me, "I am now in a natural state, and I feel wonderful. I'm doing what you talk about in Sedentary Nation, and I'm thriving."

Timeline of Decreasing Physical Movement

The Timeline emphasizes selected key points in ancient, as well as more recent, European and American history. This historical list is not intended to reflect completeness or to weigh in on the existence of a higher power. The remarks do not intend to categorize all modern conveniences as blights, blots, or banes. The abuses of modern conveniences directly contribute to vast portions of society's ills, including sedentary and dysfunctional lifestyles.

Some of the years cited are approximations. Most of the dates are commonly accepted by scholars, while some are disputed. Anthropology, history, and science are evolving fields of study.

Readers who conclude that I am guilty of "preaching in a timeline" are quite accurate. If I am able to assist you in cutting the cords of sedentism* by opening your mind and heart to our common human history of daily practices of wellness, eventually I will be preaching to the choir.

The Timeline

6 Million B.C. - Oldest known hominine fossil (Toumai) discovered in Central Africa (sources claim a date closer to 7 million B.C. than 6). These early, upright walkers are considered gatherers. Scavenging is another mode of how early, upright walkers acquired food. That means they found animals that were killed by others (or simply expired) and then grabbed what they could. Does that mean we have a hyena or vulture streak in our lineage? Undoubtedly, that may be why some of us "go ape" about garage sale deals and free stuff on clean-up days.

What this book refers to as *movement* (physical movement) is programmed into our DNA. (Some experts contend so is addiction and so is laziness.) Unlike some hibernators, most branches of the animal kingdom (humans have long been listed as part of this) lack built-in mechanisms that can keep them healthy and well without physical movement. The human tendency is to wither away (or become bloated with fat) and die without movement. For people who live off the land, days without active physical movement means there is no food—without which hunger sets in. Enough weeks without food means death. Sustenance has always been the main reason for movement. Even today we generally don't work for fun; we work to be able to afford our expenses, including groceries.

---

* U.S. physical therapists and fitness trainers have been using sedentism to convey the same meaning as sedentary lifestyle.

1.8 Million B.C. - The remains of Homo erectus hominids from this era indicate pursuits of hunting and gathering.

200,000 B.C. - Approximate appearance of Homo sapiens, as hunter-gatherers.

100,000 B.C. - DNA evidence suggests that dogs, through breeding controlled by humans, were separated from wolves around this time. They were used as hunters' helpers and are considered the first domesticated animal.

50,000 B.C. - We share the same DNA as the Homo sapiens from this era, yet we treat our bodies completely differently. Part of the human quest has been to make life easier, to minimize suffering and toil. History reveals that this hasn't always been the end result. Sedentary Nation makes the claim that lack of physical movement—including the avoidance of activities that produce huffing and puffing, increased circulation, and endorphin-type highs—directly equates to unnatural living and the breakdown of mind and body.

9,000 B.C. - Sedentary villages appear. Inhabitants domesticate animals, seeds, and plants concurrently with continued hunting and gathering. This immediately initiated social classes and long hours of work for the field workers.

Some sources put the advent of farming several thousand years ahead of the longstanding date of 9,000 B.C. which saw farming in settlements in the Fertile Crescent such as Jericho and Gobekli Tepi. A location called Ohalo II in the Sea of Galilee holds seed evidence that has been dated to 23,000 years ago. Though some writings still consider this tribal group to be hunter-gatherers.

Scientists and sociologists readily make clear that Homo sapiens have two major traits about which we should all be aware:

1. Evolution has programmed us to hold onto calories, storing them as fat, for long winters or other periods of food scarcity.

2. As a group and as individuals, we tend to focus on the immediate. We have rarely been adept long-term planners, and for that reason we have frequently not acted ecologically. Our choices have regularly destroyed our planet's systems and each other instead of working within natural, holistic living paradigms—*and planning for the future.*

Today, much of this has to do with the shortsightedness of greedy people at the top who are sponsored by hungry, greedy, and ignorant constituents.

7,000 B.C. - One of the first cities grows from a small village in Jericho, Palestine. Not counting certain empires that built large cities (for example, the Roman Empire), widespread (meaning across the planet) urbanization did not exist until the 19th century A.D. Up to that point, there was typically no way to provision large populations of city dwellers. Urbanization grew vigorously when civilizations were able to feed people who served in administrative, clerical, and ruling hierarchies, as well as those who worked in sales and production—initially workers like builders, artisans, and merchants. Eventually, factories, mills, and plants created more areas of dense population.

4,000 B.C. - Oxen are used as draft animals. At times, people were panting and sweating during daily chores, as well as travel by foot. At other times they remained still, or moved quietly, breathing softly, when they needed to sneak up on game … or while playing hide-and-seek.

500–400 B.C. - For Greeks, as revealed in their art and written records, creating beautiful human bodies meant people were more godlike. This is perhaps the first popular example of pumping iron and posing for the purpose of looking good.

General Trend of Food and Movement (Not Date-Specific)

Ready-to-eat food, including ready-cooked, is frequently connected with urbanization, but hunter-gatherers and farmer-cultivators also needed food to go—fast food. Humans are more able to perform their tasks when supplied with continual nourishment. People often think of vitamins and minerals when they think of food, and both are important. But food's most important and immediate role is to provide calories. Without calories in the system, the human engine is less able to generate movement. Lack of movement leads to starvation. Thin people starve relatively quickly. From the time of the original sedentary villages, cultivators and hunter-gatherers continue to populate the globe. Vast populations die off while others prosper. Most everyone has a physical job they are required to perform, and most jobs revolve around the acquisition, production, and delivery of food.

In the Eastern Roman Empire, children and military recruits are sent to schools to learn. Eventually, this practice leads to masses of young people being *forced into* remaining seated (a sedentary position often taken up on the ground) or standing in one general area for long periods of time. This ultimately led to providing chairs and desks to students.

Sitting at school desks inherently sets us up to accept as true that spending long durations of time seated in constricting apparatuses is normal. Some would argue an easy way to control a population is to get it sitting down and listening to repeated messages from the controlling forces. School teaching is generally based upon an approved and required curriculum (including sponsored textbooks), funded by tax dollars and overseen by government entities. School also teaches obedience to the system.

By design, today's system is, as a rule, production and consumption oriented, not liberation and discovery oriented. Intrinsically, nations are organized under unity, defense, obedience, propaganda, and control. All of this needs directors and enforcers, who, just like the masses, need to be fed, clothed, and housed. The more a hierarchy is top heavy, the more the food workers become resentful of those who are not toiling in the fields but instead hire people (enforcers, thugs, bad *hombres*) to wield whips (or withhold pay) and impose authority.

In Asia, many followed teachings inspired by Confucius, aka Master Kong, a Chinese philosopher who is said to have lived around 500 B.C. Physical movement—including tai chi, martial arts, sword practice, and holding positions—with a spiritual motivation leads the practitioner to health, focus, and moral character.

In India, a daily practice first concentrated on the spiritual side comes into use. Yoga, which means "union," was developed by Hindu priests because they saw the benefits of moving their bodies during parts of their meditation. They knew that sitting around and *just attempting to move the mind and spirit* generally produced immediate and chronic threats to wellbeing. Of some adept gurus, it is said they are able to move the energy through their body without physical movement.

Rome: 60 A.D. - Nero builds a public *gymnasium*: Greek word for "place to be naked." These were places *men* could go to train, be social, and experience intellectual stimulation. The heart, the mind, and the body were kept invigorated. Much of this took place without roofs—sunlight during the day, fresh air after sunset. Remember that ventilation and sunshine are important factors in sanitary cleanliness.

Roman citizens had long maintained their physical fitness for battle readiness. But over time, fitness subsided. Gluttony, complacency, and laziness (and even lead poisoning from pipes and utensils, among other things) increased during periods of excess, plagues, and overpopulation. The population eventually grew more unfit and the physical infrastructure (roads, buildings, aqueducts) fell into varying states of disrepair. Invaders vandalized aqueducts, thus cutting off water supplies. (The same technique, *turning off the water*, was employed by the Nazis in 1943 in the final battle in the ghetto of Warsaw.)

The Western Roman Empire eventually declined to the point of being unable to get food from the farms into the urban areas to feed the populations. The capital city of Ancient Rome once boasted 40,000 apartment units and almost 2,000 palaces. Barbaric tribes conquered Rome partly because of the physical strength and unity of the tribes, who lived mainly as hunter-gatherers while also raising domesticated cattle. Well-to-do Romans found it *inconvenient* to die for the Empire. And the poor, increasingly turning to Christianity and its promise of a paradise after death, preferred martyrdom to serving the Caesar. The result: hiring of mercenaries to take the place of the legendary Roman Legions. Alaric, the Christian barbarian king, was reportedly met at the gates of Rome by mercenaries. The rest of the story can be summed up: "Money talked, mercenaries walked."

After the gluttonous Roman civilization crumbled (476 A.D.), the lives of many returned to a survival mode where only the fittest and best cooperators survived. Roman citizens were kicked out of their condos and sent packing. They were essentially on the run. Some of these former city dwellers even became highway bandits. Others took to the fields and worked the land. If they didn't do well in working the land or stealing from those who did, they perished.

The end of the Eastern Roman Empire was not until 1453 A.D. with the conquering of Constantinople by the Seljuk Turks, or as we know them, another dark horde from the Siberian Steppes.

The Middle Ages, 6th–15th century - The early period had some populations moving away from cities. Subsistence farming eventually gave way to feudalism. The lives of the masses revolved around food. The field workers—serfs—toiled away, protected by the landowners—lords. History has shown how the wealthy would keep the workers down so that the workers would have substantial challenges in organizing into a fighting force against their *masters*. The ruling class did, however, need fit soldiers who generally came from farm-worker stock. This was a period noted for backbreaking work and wars. Conditions of harshness and endless repetition seemingly provide an indication of why humans would someday gravitate to living indoors and flipping channels.

Renaissance, 14th–17th century - It was common for the royals, the king and queen included, to recreate via dancing balls, walking, riding horses, hunting, fencing, and sex. Over the course of history, sex (not just in long-term partnership) was at times used recreationally … and still is. See your own sources or refer to the cultural phenomenon called the "hook up" and refer to the 2010 best-selling book "Sex at Dawn." Also see how the bonobos, our closest DNA relative, use sex for stress relief and to squelch communal disturbances. One 17-year-old prep school adolescent male thought it a bit strange when he was asked if he was going out on dates in 2013. "Dates are out. Today it's the hook-up. You meet them at parties or wherever. You make out and that's it. Done. You don't even exchange phone numbers. Who needs the aggravation and who has the time for all of the dinners and movies?"

1519 - The horse is reintroduced to the Americas by Cortés, Spanish conquistador. Only this time it's a big horse. Ancient North American protohorses had evolved in stature from the size of a fox to the size of a large dog before going extinct some 10,000 years prior to the European Renaissance. These mini horses had toes instead of hooves. The strong and durable Spanish-Arabic horses that did well in places like the Great Plains enabled Native American tribes to expand their territories and have more contact with European traders who gave them modern steel weapons and tools in exchange for things like tanned buffalo hides. The horse enabled native peoples to thrive for a time. The horse culture quickly became an environment where native warriors spent vast portions of their time guarding their horses as well as stealing horses from whites and from neighboring Indian tribes.

United States Modern Period, Beginning in the 1600s - Forced sedentism of Native Americans. The settlers and the governing bodies removed Indians from their traditional tribal homelands and hunting grounds and tried to force them to be sedentary farmers. Depression, alcoholism, obesity, poverty, and drug addiction became prevalent on reservations.

U.S. Late-Modern Period, 1800s–2000s - In 1800, 95 percent of Americans lived in rural areas. By 1920, due to immigration and the Industrial Revolution, some 60 percent lived in cities. In the early 1800s, 95 percent of people worked in some capacity related to growing food. Today the number is reportedly less than 5 percent.

How aerobic is the life of a cowboy? If the work of a cowboy or cowgirl has them huffing and puffing over long durations, that's an indication of aerobics. If a cowpoke is just slowly riding the property line watching the stock, his activity is deficient in significant physical exertion.

Neck and spine pain plagues sedentary humans. Maintaining a head-down position puts tremendous stress on the body and is easily evidenced in postures assumed for reading, writing, laptop, and beadwork. Many four-legged animals have a strong nuchal ligament (aka paddywhack as in ..."With a knick-knack, paddywhack, give a dog a bone. This old man came rolling home"). Grazing animals like deer, moose, and horses have biomechanical structures and musculature to support the weight of their heads. Evolution made them masters of the horizontal-leaning head position. Human necks (and the integrity of our upright anatomy) aren't built for grazing ... or surfing on low-angled digitized screens all day—and evening.

The African-American slaves are freed from slave masters. At first, some of the freed slaves are given land, often referred to by the phrase "40 acres and a mule." When this practice ended, a great deal of land was given back to whites, forcing countless African Americans to work as sharecroppers, which spelled more poverty and subservience for them. From 1890 to 1970, in what is known as the Great Migration, more than 6 million African-Americans left the South and settled in the North. For African-Americans, urban populations grew, as did sedentary lifestyles.

A recent report said that African-Americans spent more time with TV and digital devices than any other ethnicity.[14] Latinos were listed in second place. In the U.S., these two groups suffer the highest per capita percentages of obesity, asthma, heart problems, and poverty.

1828 - The iron horse (steam locomotive) is developed. Tracks laid at Baltimore Harbor and, in 1830, in New York. The train is arguably one of the most comfortable of all modes of transportation when interiors are spacious and tracks are kept smooth. Sedentism is reduced since passengers can move about with relative safety. On longer trips, passengers can even step off the train at periodic stops for stretch breaks. As witnessed recently, some actively stretch their legs; others stand around and smoke.

1845 - The Police Gazette is founded in New York City. One of the first American tabloids, it enjoyed tremendous success based on creating a readership ripe for stories and illustrations of scandal, obscenity, and gossip. Long published on pink newspaper stock, it created a following of readers intrigued to read about the lives of actresses, chorus girls, and prize fighters, as well as other stories deemed of potential interest to the curious masses. It used sensationalism and yellow journalism better than most of the papers of its time and was instrumental in creating a pop culture that had readers spending increasing stretches of time preoccupied with the lives of others. Degradation and decrepitude normally follow when citizens spend more time following the lives of the famous and infamous than they do taking care of themselves, their families, and their community.

1854 - The Otis elevator is installed at the World's Fair in New York City. The construction of tall buildings necessitates new modes of conveyance for humans and supplies.

1896 - The escalator debuts at Old Iron Pier at Coney Island, New York. It was developed, in part, to move people through congested areas.

1890s–1960 - Dance halls could be found in towns small and large across the United States and Western Europe. Dance halls were a place for people to congregate, dance to live music, and meet new friends. The Savoy in Harlem during the 1930s has been called the first truly integrated building in the United States ... for both dancers and musicians. Dancing is an unwinding celebration creating, on its positive side, an opportunity to bring out the best in people. As a regular activity starting from youth, large numbers of people developed their skills and became proficient. It was *cool* to get in on the fun.

1899–1900 - The first American truck was developed by a team headed by engineer Louis Semple Clarke and released for sale by the Pittsburgh Motor Vehicle Company. Trucks, trains, and ships allow for distance shipping of nearly everything, including food. Truck driving is one of the classic sedentary jobs and has long caused its share of pronounced physical disabilities. The restaurants at truck stops have traditionally provided heavy, greasy fare, and the chance to use the cigarette machine.

1900s - An exodus from farms continued to satisfy the worker needs of the Industrial Revolution and war efforts. Untold numbers left farms with hopes of a better life. They already knew that farming was extremely difficult work and in no way promised land ownership.

(The following is one of the most startling facts uncovered while writing Sedentary Nation. This encapsulates the overriding theme of man's complacency with the paradigm of profit and control in trumping wellness and doing the right thing.) Because of the almost inconceivable reason that six to nine months of storage life for milled flour wasn't long enough for bread industrialists, wheat flour is bleached with potentially harmful chemicals (including chlorine dioxide) in order to keep it from going rancid. The modern era preserving process removes or depletes many of the good things that wheat bread originally provided, including unsaturated fatty acids, proteins, vitamins, and trace minerals (especially magnesium, selenium, and chromium). These things may not matter to consumers once they are easily convinced that "it's all about taste." The current health food movement veers away from low-cost, nutrient deficient food in favor of better nutrition. The experts all agree the end result is improved overall health and wellbeing—ultimately the lower cost way to live.

1906 - Upton Sinclair writes what became the new century's classic American work of muckraking. It was censored and only its softer rewrite—which toned down the harshness of the work conditions—was permitted to be published. "The Jungle," a work of historically accurate fiction, exposes abuses of human labor, examples of horrible treatment of animals during slaughtering, and atrocious health hazards related to meat processing. Its popular success provoked immediate reform. Once again, reforms are drastically needed in the new millennium. According to the 2009 documentary "Food Inc.," in 1972, there were roughly 50,000 FDA inspections of meat and poultry processing plants versus 9,200 inspections in 2006. Much of this is due to lesser government oversight of food corporations. Part of this is due to consolidation by corporate giants—there are far fewer plants.

1913–1918 - WWI is the first major war to institute a petroleum-powered, mechanized military. Still, it could be considered an old-school war. Reports claim that 6 to 8 million horses died in the conflict. The muddy trenches (and virtual lack of sanitation), and dead humans and horses, made for a toxic and sometimes sedentary field of war. One 4-month stretch of the war resulted in more than 1 million casualties, with only six miles of land changing hands between the opposing warriors. Some records show that British soldiers were sometimes fed rations of beef for breakfast; Americans in the trenches were known to take a morning meal of coffee, donuts, and cigarettes. The pancreas, teeth and gums, and our other markers of wellness (including the bowels) certainly don't respond well to the American trench breakfast diet. In this case, meat provided a more stable blood sugar level than carbohydrates, poison, and junk.

1915 - The beginning of what obesity researcher Dr. Richard Lustig, M.D., calls "The Coca-Cola Conspiracy." The expanding container sizes of soft drinks parallels the supersizing of Westerners. Sugar, he emphatically states, is causing obesity: 1916, 6.5-oz. glass contour bottle; 1955, 10-oz. bottle; 1960, 12-oz. cans; 1988, 44-oz. huge cups; 1992, 20-oz. plastic bottle; 2011, smaller plastic bottles introduced because, "Americans are counting both their calories and their pennies."[15] Caffeine is a diuretic, which makes you urinate good water. That plus the sodium (salt) in cola makes you thirsty and makes you drink more. The more salt in cola, the more sugar is needed to mask the salt. Dr. Lustig says, "They [Coca-Cola and other soft drink companies who follow this model] knew exactly what they were doing."

Ask yourselves if PepsiCo knows what it's doing when it sponsors playgrounds around the world that feature product logos and images.

1916 - White Castle opens its first location in Wichita, Kansas, and becomes known as the first hamburger chain. When it opened its doors, it only charged 5¢ per burger. Cheap and convenient fast food is a significant part of our sedentary world.

1919 - The gasoline-powered lawnmower is first manufactured in the United States, but homeowners continue to use push-reel lawnmowers and scythes because they work well and burn calories rather than hard-earned wages.

If you were regular folk, your lawn didn't have to be perfect. You didn't normally have to keep up with the Joneses. You just needed a place for your kids to play and perhaps for you to invite some friends and family over for a Sunday afternoon outdoor meal.

1920s - Radio networks begin broadcasting. Listeners are not required to sit idly. They can still move their bodies and accomplish things while being entertained or informed, *though some just stared at the box*. Terrific scripts, directors, actors, and sound effects permitted listeners' imaginations to come up with their own images for the popular radio shows. Some argue that the mind was experiencing richer engagement without the use of any visual screens. Instead of fancy photographic visual effects—and the viewer's amazement at *what they [the photographic producers] can do*—radio permits the brain to do one thing it does superbly, create its own images. Look what it can do.

1930s - Howard Johnson's pioneers franchised restaurants with standardized menus and marketing. Since the food is the same in any of their restaurants, you get what you pay for whether you're in downtown Queens or on the outskirts of Alameda. Food becomes as standardized as toilet paper. Fast forward to today's typical supermarkets where your purchasing is limited to three main apple types—all uniform, none with any marks, stamped with a label, coated in wax—that were all sprayed with various chemicals while on the tree. One spray causes them to ripen and another to drop to the ground.

1940s and beyond - World War II brings an extraordinary mechanized war effort. The desire and need for automation and mechanization begins to permeate all areas of life, including lawn mowing, which, more and more, is handled with power mowers. The countdown to microwave ovens begins. Four decades later, they will become standard issue appliances in mid-range new construction. Homes increasingly become electronics warehouses that have residents being bombarded by what some consider hazardous EMFs.

1951 - TV networks broadcast from coast to coast and the visual medium replaces radio as the dominant home entertainment medium. TV increases sedentary living and almost instantly becomes *the major addiction* that leads to a sedentary lifestyle. Nearly every family with a parking spot owns or has access to one automobile. Urban and suburban grandmothers may still walk to the market and church, but it becomes increasingly unlikely that their adult children will.

Up until the time that TV became a preferred pastime, kids who weren't working a job would play games, frequently outdoors, even in inclement weather. Some games were competitive; some were just for kicks. A senior citizen had tears in his eyes in 1987 when he told me, "Kids today are missing out. We used to play football in the fall, basketball in the winter, and baseball in the spring. I don't get them with this TV flipping." What he didn't get was the term "addiction"—addiction to an indoor, sedentary lifestyle.

20th century - Couches, previously reserved for those of privileged wealth, are now within financial reach of the masses. With more disposable income than their predecessors, the working class can afford couches for the first time in history. Couch potatoes (of all classes) are, in part, formed when people become excessively and unproductively sedentary. In most cases, the TV is the main couch-centric pastime. Since it's hard to pull away from the boob tube—for some, impossible—it clearly has become a powerful addiction.

Positive pursuits like resting and relaxing after work or school, reading and improving education, and communing with family and friends, are placed on the back burner. Instead of actively recreating or getting some needed rest, a group some have termed *lemmings* tune in for more stimulation (not just quality programming, but the mind-numbing news, flashy imagery, and invasive sound) from the TV. In the 1970s, comedian George Carlin imitated a home-based woman who had to cut her phone conversation short, "... because my stories [soap operas] are coming on."

Without having time to quiet their minds, many remain worn out—*wired* by unhealthful options and choices. Some writers criticize the 20th century, whose worship of pop culture creates a dumbing down of society. An entire population, many of whom witnessed the backbreaking work of their family's elders, is cajoled into further sedentism and hyper consumerism. TV, whose language is often based on a less than ninth-grade education, leads this trend. Media writers, once taught to cater to eighth-grade levels, eventually have to stoop even lower to reach their average audience.* Instead of creating a wiser electorate, the Age of Information creates a dearth of common sense.

It could be argued that the more TV you watch, the less engaged you are in true contemplation, critical thinking, and problem solving. (Watching a program for enjoyment, learning, or both, and discussing it or reflecting on it before flipping to another one seems of higher intellectual and interactive gain than mere channel surfing.) Devoid of knowledge about how to live off the land, subjected to mass campaigns of idiocy in TV programming and commercials, people become subject to excessive behavior. Living a simple life away from malls, bars, and hair salons doesn't correlate to ignorance—just the opposite. Keeping up with the Joneses and never being satisfied is an offshoot of mass consumerism. The 20th century's extreme capitalism in a growing economy was made possible by extreme consumerism. The spread of this image—keeping up with the Joneses and the families Westerners got to know via TV programming—contributes

---

* This is an email reply I received from a scholar who has worked in a variety of fields including journalism and the military. The concept of media writing for eighth-grade level educations was not easy to find, but I remember being taught that in high school. "This knowledge is something you learn when working within the journalism world. As far as I know it is not 'written' anywhere. But every newsroom, TV newsroom, moviemaker, etc., knows the literacy level at which to aim the product. A college professor once said to me, 'Write your paper as if you are trying to educate an eighth-grade 14-year-old about a topic of which he has no knowledge.' I had known for years about the general literacy level of the newspapers that crossed my desk while in the business. That literacy level was the occasion of much hilarity when it came to writing for college educated commanding officers with some fairly sharp critical thinking skills."

to extreme sedentism. Extreme sedentism programs us more to buy things on impulse or to fix ourselves.

To promote literacy, Margaret McNamara, former teacher and the wife of Robert McNamara—JFK's secretary of defense and one of the brightest minds (but not most altruistic) in Big Power at the time—gathers a team of volunteers. In 1966, Mrs. McNamara and her volunteers began the program of donating new and used books to young school children. Reading Is Fundamental has suffered due to budget cuts. The dumbing down of society gains strength.

The 20th century Western Fitness Pioneers, Bernarr McFadden, Paige Palmer, Dr. Kenneth Cooper, Bonnie Prudden, Jack LaLanne, George Leonard, Jim Fixx, Covert Bailey, and others, lay the groundwork for the modern fitness movement. They all were concerned with the same issue—getting their adherents moving and exercising.

1950s - America is home to a growing beer culture. Beer companies sponsor football games, and countless viewers sit idly while packing in the calories from beer, soft drinks, and greasy foods like pizza. (Mentioning this here is not to categorically suggest that fermented alcohol is bad or that good quality pizza doesn't have its place.) Over time, sports TV becomes a powerful addiction. It will become more common for citizens to watch others doing movement activities than to be enjoying outdoor recreation themselves. Some may call this laziness, but it's more correctly termed an addiction that increases over time.

1953 - Swanson's TV Dinner is introduced. Americans welcome the faithful meal of turkey, stuffing, gravy, and cherry tart patterned after an original New England Thanksgiving meal. The notion of frozen dinners is not a bad one, but an overreliance on prefabricated, processed food means fewer nutrients, more preservatives, and less pride in preparing food from scratch.

Juicing (using steroids) helps make some athletes superstars. In 1954, after watching his team break world records, the Soviet weightlifting coach tells American team physician, Dr. John Ziegler, that the Soviet team uses steroids and other concoctions to boost performance. This reportedly led to the introduction of performance-enhancing substances in American sports and other forms of *cheating* with drugs and blood doping. The prevalence of doping had gained momentum among cyclists in the Tour de France, which has had revelations of doping since the Tour began in 1903. The need to perform almost impossible feats of strength and endurance was predominantly induced by sponsors of the Tour who wanted winners coupled with racers desiring to earn a living and eventually achieve fame and fortune.[16]

1956 - During Eisenhower's presidency, the President's Council on Physical Fitness is organized as a response to unfit American children (as compared to European children).

1957 - Scientists develop a way to turn corn's sucrose into high fructose. It will take corporations 20 years to drop that bomb on society. By the 1990s, high fructose corn syrup is a leading ingredient in a wide range of products including juices and cereals marketed to children. A number of scientists also consider high fructose corn syrup a gateway drug (one that leads to other drugs). Eventually, even ascorbic acid—found in most of our vitamin C pills and powders—is chemically produced from corn syrup.

1960s - Public dance halls are replaced by private discothèques (roller rinks and the disco movement came in the '70s).

Counting their early appearances in Europe, the Beatles only tour for a handful of years before deciding to stay in the studio to record. Plenty of rock musicians binge and party, yet generally stay slim.* Most of their maintained slimness may have been because this was an era before severe sedentism, corn syrup, large portions, and high-calorie mushy food.

In their younger days, music icons like the Big Bopper (210 lbs; d. 1959) and Fats Domino were neither big nor fat in comparison with heavy singers of more recent decades. Elvis' transformation from '50s heartthrob to the '70s bloated addict is hard to forget. Vast numbers of the late 20th-century and early 21st-century rock stars have trouble with excessive pounds, even as young people—some examples being Bobby Brown, Brittany Spears, and Christina Aguilera. The 1960's performers in the group The Temptations were just as good at moving to the beat as they were at singing—all members of this Motown group were relatively lean in the 1960s. (Some will argue that youthful age is the reason and that metabolism slows with age. If your metabolism slows, do you think it sensible to become less active and more gluttonous?)

The 1960s show a sharp rise in inflammation-related diseases. Some scientists include arthritis, asthma, cancer, Alzheimer's, heart disease, and chronic pain in this list and consider the rise in EMFs combined with ungrounded lifestyles as direct causes.

---

* In the year before his death, Doors' lead singer Jim Morrison looked atrocious: pudgy and sickly due to binging on alcohol and drugs. It's not accurate to say that he looked 10 or 20 years older than his 27 years. People don't necessarily look more atrocious as they age. I also heard an interview with Doors' keyboardist Ray Manzarek in which he praises his friend but lightly laments the fact that Jim Morrison wasted so much of his potential creative time by going out to bars with hangers on. "He should have spent that time writing and creating. He was too easily convinced to go out and drink and talk."

Because of walking barefoot or in leather-soled shoes, people were grounded to the Earth in prior generations. (Outdoor animals still are.) Some scientists suggest this played a role in neutralizing free radicals and instantaneously reset our voltage to the same level as the Earth's. The 1960s ushered in rubber-soled shoes and wall-to-wall-carpeted homes, which substantially reduced human grounding.[17]

1970s - In the modern era, the 1970s mark a big line in the sand for the downward spiral of socioeconomic trends in the West. Sociologist Ira Goldstein points out that the early 1970s ring in the beginning of the decline in the U.S. standard of living largely caused by a decline in domestic productivity. Production goes overseas and across borders leading to less of a demand for skilled and unskilled laborers at home. This also leads to more geographical and income distance between the classes, including a decline in real income for middle income levels. Depression and anxiety lead to further couch potato syndrome, addiction (including endless caloric intake), and sedentism.

1973 - The first Miller Lite beer TV commercial featuring football players is produced, a sign that accumulation of excess fat had begun to take hold in Western society, especially in the lives of the sedentary viewers.

1977 - Some 20 years after its initial development, high fructose corn syrup is produced and marketed by large corporations with deep pockets and strong influence. Is their influence the reason the U.S. government imposed tariffs and quotas on sugar imports (which made their corn product the much cheaper option) in the same year? You bet it is! Greedy, bleepin', shortsighted, controlling corporate and political buffoons.

1977 - A big year for *huge* Federal government snafus. Here's another one: the U.S. government sets its policy to adopt the low-fat diet. The adopted philosophy is called the diet-heart hypothesis and, according to one body of research, incorrectly correlates heart disease predominantly with LDL levels (these levels may not be as vital a concern as we have been told since the body and especially the brain need cholesterol).

The argument against the flawed government policy favors diets higher in percentages of protein and fat and lower in carbs. It especially says to avoid those carbohydrates that tend to spike insulin production. Some easy examples are breads, pastas, processed grains, and sugars. The high-protein diet would be better termed the "low-carb balanced diet." .

This protocol calls for eating some foods that contain saturated fatty acids. This might include coconut oil, nuts and seeds, avocados, animal fat, and butter. It should exclude heavily processed transfats like margarine. The saturated fatty acids are sometimes deemed harmful, since they increase total lipids. Scientific experiments have shown these diets raise HDL (think "H" for "Healthy," aka the good transporters of cholesterol) even more. Studies have come to conclusions on both sides of the higher fat, lower fat argument.

Some consider the low-fat diet the really big coup and turning point, and arguably the big hinge toward pancreatic malfeasance, obesity, brain disorders like dementia, and other downturns in wellness. The studies available in 1977, including pre-World War II German research, might just as easily have caused the U.S. government to adopt a diet of low-sugar (low simple carbs), low-sodium foods with limited processing and low contamination. Instead, the dietary practices of Americans were filled with all of these banes. Waxing revisionist, look what these choices, together with the pandemic of sedentism, have done. (Ask an older, fitness-oriented physician—one who is a now a senior citizen—how she feels about the change in her patients' physiques over her years in practice in the late 20th century.)

Adopting a dietary practice of three square meals a day was an additional big turning point in the modern diet. If they were not affluent, your family likely took up this custom somewhere in the past three generations. Residents of thinner, wine drinking France still tend to do little in the way of breakfast.

Besides eating more frequently, eating later at night became prevalent over the past three generations. Late dinners followed advances in illumination. Originally credited to flames, as in lamp and candle lighting, light was eventually handled by electric bulbs. For hunter-gathers with predators lurking and insects crawling, later eating is not as practical. It's not simply a matter of eating in peace, it's also important to shed light on the task of cleaning up. If you didn't dispose of the food scraps and get your utensils and your face and hands spic and span, insects and rodents could find a free meal—nibbling at your chin. How appreciative would you be of a bear's claws slashing through your teepee?

I mentioned the hunter-gatherer who goes out to hunt early in the morning. That happened. But it's also true that if the tribe had been fed well the previous day, or if their bodily structures were filled out with sufficient fat, they willingly and habitually lived off their fat stores. That goes even for those who were scrawny. People without much fat still have to live of their personal body's limited fat stores. Imagine a band of hungry hunters, accompanied by their tribe, embarking on a trek to catch up to distant herds. This periodic lack of food essentially mandated fasting, not to mention significant and regular long-duration exercise.

This notion of three meals or more per day is a modern—and some would say erroneous—view of how we are supposed to handle our calorie intake and usage. Eating is an enjoyable pastime and a welcome break; however, it has become an addiction. Nearly all of us are ill adept at living off our fat stores. So many of us eat far too frequently and consume too many simple carbohydrates. This prevents our metabolic system from effectively tapping our fat stores. On the contrary, this is a recipe for increasing the capacity of fat stores.

1970s - Higher percentages of people begin to show the unhealthful signs of sedentary lifestyles coupled with high-calorie diets. Kids who still actively play through their high school years don't show much roundness but inactive adults do—their belt sizes grow a few notches. The term "health nut" is at times used pejoratively in criticizing people who take care of their bodies. As a health push emerges, health food stores and vitamins (better termed supplements) gain popularity.

1980s - Increased prevalence of both desk and couch potatoes. Desk potatoes are known to sit in cubicles, private offices, open floor plans, or behind counters. A better option would be to have them doing some work standing at a high desk or counter and some sitting on a high, adjustable-position stool with an attached footrest. These people, as well as the rest of Americans, use fast food and junk food on a regular basis; some slug it down daily.

The Age of Video and Information helps make short attention spans even shorter, which makes people more subject to deception and addiction. The Baby Boomers are known to prize youthfulness and money, while resenting their immobile, sedentary lifestyles—and ultimately, themselves. Unlike the nuclear family units of the 1950s, fragmented families became the norm. Especially noticeable in the cultures of white and black American families is that the grandparents are recurrently no longer part of the family unit—unless they are called upon to be parents again. "Everyone wants their space," is an oft-used adage.

The nuclear family detonates in divorce, and 30-year careers are cut short due to changes in economics and human resource strategies. For example, at-will employees can and are hired and fired at will; pension plans are reduced, pillaged by predators, or eliminated. This runs concurrently with the notion of everyone having a personal psychological counselor. The hardy souls from rural America and the Great Depression—both of whose ranks were physically and mentally pooped out at the end of an average day—are replaced by droves of wired people who stay up late. Cable TV provides an incredible number of options, 24 hours a day.

Large fitness centers populate America. With fluorescent lights; central ventilation; black rubber floor coverings; chemical, germ-fighting, cleansing sprays; Velcro and vinyl; and tinted windows or no windows; there is a total disconnect from nature and the outdoors. From the outside, mega fitness centers might look like any other box store. Diana Ross created a hit with lyrics that went, "I want muscles …"

"If you didn't belong to a gym," a friend says about this era, "there was something wrong with you."

Over the history of the known world, people generally would rise with or before the sunrise and bed down within a few hours of sunset. Twentieth-century inventions create large numbers of people who remain awake until late at night. People are fatigued, yet they experience sleep disorders. Indoor lifestyles demand electrical lights, which produce EMF radiation and produce no vitamin D. This combined with non-physical jobs and at-home access to entertainment boxes and high sugar foods and beverages continues to generate stress and compromise health.

In the late 1990s, it's not uncommon to find each adult member of a family with a personal automobile or to see each family member with a personal TV. Driveways become parking lots and bedrooms become havens of screen-time entertainment. People—especially and ironically kids—are spending significant amounts of time indoors, plugged in to noise and imagery—and canned laughter and crime updates. Video games like Grand Theft Auto, which feature violent themes, become popular.

Sleep-related problems are largely sourced in the lack of physical work and play, the lack of vitamin D, abnormal mela-tonin levels, the stress of daily living, the stress medications that disrupt sleep patterns, and atrocious diets, which, among other things, create highly unstable blood sugar levels. This leaves adults thinking there is something wrong with them. Elder generations are not spending time side by side, working and recreating with the younger generations, besides the occasional visit or phone call. When you need wisdom, help, or someone to listen, "who you gonna call?" Or talk to ... the counselor, the bartender, the palm reader, the psychiatrist, the spiritual leader or, in the new millennium, the life coach? "Somebody's got to listen to me!"

1990s - Vast numbers of people of all ages in America become supersized. At home, dinner plates and glassware become increasingly larger. Still, plenty of people get seconds and thirds just as they did with the smaller plates used in the earlier, more active decades. Motorized mobility scooters, originally invented for disabled people, now haul around the self-inflicted and junk-food-inflicted rolls of fat belonging to the dysfunctional supersized and the morbidly obese. Experts consider many of the obese to be genetically and emotionally predisposed to obesity. For both adults and children, there is an increasing prevalence of the following conditions: diabetes, obesity, and asthma. A growing number of school-age kids carry their own prescription steroidal inhalers. The field of individual and family psychological counseling gathers more steam.

Mega churches—some as large as college campuses—flourish. Part of their growth is based on the capability to fill in for some of what used to be provided by the greater family, neighborhood, and village. Vast numbers of churches of all sizes have meetings and activities going on throughout the day and evening. Churches grow in size and scope. No longer just sanctuaries for worship with meeting halls, many churches were to grow into family centers and learning centers. Churches offer diverse options, including English as a Second Language (ESL) and computer classes, daycare, crisis intervention, senior yoga, job training, marriage counseling, and addiction meetings.

The home-cooked, American meat-and-potatoes diet of old was originally patterned after a European—not Mediterranean—ancestry. Meat and potatoes is bumped aside by the popular dishes of pasta and cheese, which typically mean excessive calories. Such dishes include carbs high on the glycemic index as well as factory-farmed animal products. For convenience and taste, people purchase and serve the highly processed, junk cheeses and pre-made mac-and-cheese offerings. Before the doping and feedlot raising of cows, the original meat-and-potatoes diet may not have been perfect, but it was arguably a better choice than the boxed food that followed. Remember, the original European-American immigrants vigorously moved their bodies for their physical jobs and tasks and needed sufficient and long-lasting calories.

Both the pasta-and-cheese and pizza diets dump lots of sugar calories and oils into the body very quickly. A diet of roughage and fiber-filled vegetables and protein and fat-rich meat takes much more human-body processing time since these ingredients need to be chewed and broken down. Even a salad with carrots and radishes takes a fair amount of chewing. Pasta and melted cheese go down with far fewer chews (as few as two or three), making meals almost swallowable. This equates to excessive calories being consumed and in the bloodstream in a much shorter period of time. Many experts consider these diets less than optimum in nutritional value. Pasta is high in carbs and cheese contains the milk sugar, lactose. Most of the harm is done when we overdo them. It's hard not to overdo them when you start out as a child and never learn the importance of nutrition or how to prepare healthful meals.

The Internet, home video games, and 24-hour cable TV (eventually beamed by satellite) have people clicking away on digital devices because, "Life itself has become boring ..." Attention spans grow even shorter.

Policymakers and parents demand more academic rigor—in some schools, P.E. and recess get reduced and even eliminated. Teachers are singled out for many of the problems in education.

Years later, teachers and districts will categorically be singled out in the much-criticized 2001 Act of Congress program No Child Left Behind. Kids, young adults, and their parents spend increasing spans of time in seated positions.

Years later, in the craze of smartphones and text messaging, an athletic teacher would tell me, "Young people's dexterity is superb, as long as you are talking about their hands."

1995 - Doritos gives an enduring Christmas present to Spain. In December, the Doritos brand is introduced there. A Spanish medical marketing consultant told me, "Before this time, we customarily ate traditional Spanish dinners, often while watching soccer games. Essentially, *tapas* or a main course and a salad were the meal. The goal of Doritos' makers [and the other snack makers as well] was to convince consumers that it was the hip thing to do ... eat snacks while watching TV. It didn't take much convincing. The foods are tasty and addicting. This meant we Spanish started with junk food and soda or beer during the games and then did our best to eat the dinner that had already been prepared. That meant we consumed lots of calories over a two- or three-hour period."

In the 1990s, worldwide snack food and fast food consumption climbs appreciably higher. Recent revenues were listed at $330 billion for snack foods and $500 billion for fast foods. Some analysts expect growth of these industries to continue.

2000s - The field of wellness takes on problems of health, diet, and inactivity. But it faces challenge in the new generation of people who are accustomed to seeking instantaneous rewards in the fast-paced, image-conscious world of short attention spans and ubiquitous convenience food. Body art, including piercings and teeth grillz with bling, as well as multiple tattoos, become vogue for a wide segment of young and middle-aged people. For many in the new generation of young men, a new movement of tattoos, smoking cigarettes, vaping, trendy hairstyles, muscles (including six-pack abs and sculpted pecs), and sexiness seems to take precedence over athletics and physical recreation, the learning of craftsmanship, and the practice of general wellness. Plastic surgery and Botox aren't just for drooping adults; young people fill out the practitioner's schedule as well. Growing percentages of high school girls are getting breast augmentation and a growing percentage of boys are getting breast reduction. One source stated that the number of breast augmentations per year in the under 18-year-old crowd rose nearly six times, to 7,882 from 1,326, over a 10-year period ending in 2007.[18]

Diet books reach record sales. The low-carb revolution causes food companies to offer low-carb products, including low-carb pizza and low-carb pasta. Sales of books by Dr. Robert Atkins (who died in 2003) reach 20 million copies. People are desperate to lose weight. Soon detractors from the low-carb craze publish reports that claim the diet is unnatural, doesn't work, and may cause harm. According to the reports from some of the highly touted physicians and researchers who come out against the low-carb diet, people have been once again duped!

The year before Dr. Atkins dies, journalist Gary Taubes publishes a momentous article in the New York Times Magazine, "What if It's All Been a Big Fat Lie?" This article was a catalyst in reinvigorating the diet debate. Through vigilant research and writing, Taubes' is able to resurrect historic studies that had been mostly forgotten by the mainstream dietary pundits. (Some of the marketers and producers of corn syrup, wheat, and corn who have long influenced national policy as well as the various designs of the federal food pyramids, had probably hoped the studies would continue to remain dormant.) Taubes' work attempts to provide more evidence that high-carb diets—sugar—are instrumental in causing us to become fat and obese.

The studies he cites show that hormones, including insulin, cause our fat cells to store more triglycerides and make us fatter as we continue to insatiably consume food that is easily converted to sugar.

What Taubes and others call Endocrinology 101, shows that many are predisposed to obesity by individual biology and chemistry. These so-called fat people crave and consume high-carb products— soda, juices, beer, breads, cakes, rice, and pasta. An insulin-resistant person is unable to process sugars. The normal person who is not yet insulin resistant has to beware sugar intake. If this non-diabetic individual continues to consume excessive sugar, their system may revolt.

This could cause them prediabetes or one of the categories of diabetes which could leave them unable to properly metabolize sugars. The individual's biochemistry has to do something with all of this sugar so it converts it to fat and dumps more and more fat molecules into a person's already burgeoning fat cells. Like compressed air into a balloon, more and more comes in, causing the balloon to grow. In the human body, more fat means the fat cells fill up and expand.

One study featured 811 participants; 62 percent women, 38 percent men. This two-year study found that four different diets all achieved similar results in terms of weight and waistline reduction and improved health. The participants followed strict diets based on four different groups, which were separated based on varying percentages of fat, protein, and carbohydrates. The key to the study's good results was a 750-calorie reduction daily diet. No daily intake was below 1200 calories. Thus, in this case, it wasn't as much what percentages of calories came from what food group, but the total number of calories. The participants also did moderate exercise and consumed calories considered more healthful. As far as weight loss, in this particular study, those who participated in counseling sessions did better.[19] A major criticism of studies like these is the accountability of the dieting subjects—people can and do cheat. Though you may continue to hear varying success stories with different dietary regimes, intellectually speaking, there's nothing wrong with trying a particular diet and seeing if it works for you. Again, your health history should be considered and your health should be monitored.

Increasing sales of popular books and documentaries show historical and behind-the-scenes looks at wellness, including diet, food sources, food conglomerates, and human addiction. Some notables to mention: "Food Inc.," "Fast Food Nation," "The Future of Food," "Supersize Me," "Healthy at 100," "The China Study," "The Omnivore's Dilemma," and "May I Be Frank."

Parents and educators are concerned with how to properly raise children in the age of digital, sugar, and short attention spans. Considerable numbers of books and documentaries are released in attempts to inform people of the best methods for interacting with special needs children.

The world is also full of special needs adults. Who doesn't have special needs? In 2001, Robert J. MacKenzie publishes his book "Setting Limits with Your Strong-Willed Child: Eliminating Conflict by Establishing Clear, Firm, and Respectful Boundaries." It's not only a book that can help parents and teachers, but all of us might pay heed to establishing respectful boundaries in our own relationships and in regard to our own behavioral shortcomings, including inclinations toward digital overload, poor diet, and excessive work. Again, it's not only young people who have trouble controlling impulses. We all need to realize how our emotions and brain chemistry are triggered by sensations, memories, and images.

Pack your bags if you have been diagnosed with pancreatic cancer, which has historically had a 5 percent survival rate and, as a rule, is considered to be directly related to lifestyle—especially boozing. It takes about 20 years to generate its symptoms. That means that by the time it is diagnosed, it's normally too late. For 95 percent of those with this diagnosis, the trip leaves very soon.

Functional training, Pilates, Zumba, CrossFit, P90X, spinning, Egoscue, cardio kickboxing, kettle bells, Body Boot Camp, Super Slow, Body By Science, qi gong, yoga and other parts of the fitness and physical activity movement are popularized in the United States. These are generally considered purposeful physical activities with goals including getting in shape and promoting balance or union of mind, body, and spirit. Many of the popular sports of our recent past are generally recreational in nature while still providing a competitive component. Think of racquet sports such as tennis, squash, badminton, racquetball, ping pong, as well as other sports like softball, touch football, soccer, and golf.

These activities aren't taken up to put money in your pocket or food on your table—as in farming or hunting-gathering—nor do they get you to your next destination as in walking or running. But they are some of the practical answers to the crisis of inactivity and lack of mind-body connection. The group classes also provide zing from what is known as the group dynamic; they also provide camaraderie.

"Dancing with the Stars" and "The Biggest Loser" TV programs showcase movement that sedentary viewers can watch as they sit, casually enjoying how other people are burning calories. There's hope that the show also motivates viewers to take up physical movement.

Some pay-per-view watchers reserve the evening to watch physical combat. The Ultimate Fighting Champion (UFC) and other limited-rules fighting competitions replace boxing as the big draw on cable TV. This causes enrollment in martial arts to soar. Record numbers of new schools open to offer grappling arts. These activities hearken back to ancient human practices as well as those of animals like tigers and bears. Tigers and bears grapple from an early age and do so their entire lives to settle disputes without fatality and to keep up their physical skills. Cable TV programmers respond in a big way. They sense their viewers want to see more devastation and mayhem than the grappling arts provide. The answer is found in the sometimes bloody and gory mixed martial arts cage fighting programs (like the UFC), which cater to the bloodlust as did the gladiatorial fights during the Roman Empire. At times, ancient gladiatorial bouts got the bloodlust ramped up so high that men would leave the arena and terrorize the town and each other (a la European soccer hooligans). This bloody bedlam was eased by lining the areas near the arena's exits with prostitutes—in some cases, thousands of them.

2005 - Dr. T. Colin Campbell, a 50-year government researcher and policy insider, publishes "The China Study." He boldly points out, "Most nutrition and health information is very misleading. It is no coincidence that we now have a medical care crisis which is very expensive and which compromises the quality of life for millions of Americans and others living on a Western-style diet." Dr. Campbell is also a long-time recreational runner who grew up on a dairy farm in Virginia. Some practicing physicians claim that it's not even a study, just a collection of untested observations. They criticize "The China Study," especially its vegetarian claims citing our history as scavengers and hunters as well as recent nutritional science. Despite the debate, no one seems to be saying to avoid fresh vegetables and living a balanced life. (Can you see a pie fight in the making?) A detractor to vegetarian philosophy is Dr. Loren Cordain, author of "The Paleo Diet," who states, "When I initially became involved in evolutionary nutrition, I knew that common diseases of civilization like hypertension, high cholesterol, and cardiovascular diseases could be reduced or totally prevented by maintaining a contemporary Paleo diet," which in part means getting some of our dietary protein and fat from safe, unprocessed meat.

2008 - The movie "WALL-E" grosses $23 million on its opening day. Walk-in theatres grossing billions of dollars are filled by increasing numbers of supersized people who have atrocious eating and exercise habits. They spend money... lots of money. They spend it not only on tickets but also on the junk-food offerings at the cinema.

2009 - President Obama signs healthcare reform bills into law. The original bills only earmark $1 billion for Wellness and Prevention out of a total health budget predicted to exceed $1 trillion.

2010 - Revenues of fast food providers approach $200 billion on U.S. sales alone, which is not even close to the gross needs of the U.S. health budget. Revenues of pharmaceutical companies (which also own supplementation companies) may now exceed

$1 trillion in worldwide sales.

2011 - Jack LaLanne, a gifted motivator, beloved pioneer of fitness, gyms, juicing, and a healthy lifestyle, dies at age 96. He is the answer to the question posed earlier regarding the famous chin-up champ who is buried in Forest Lawn Cemetery in Los Angeles. He remained positive in his approach to wellness and never gave up on us. Fitness and wellness pioneer Bonnie Prudden outlives Jack by a few months, also dying at age 96.

Tony Horton's P90X become a top-selling series of fitness DVDs. His infomercial manager, Carl Daikeler, proclaims, "Whoever succeeds at making the living room an effective place to get fit is going to be a billionaire."

2012 and beyond - In the modern era, a significant portion of medical-center training and medical-industry schooling have historically been based on teaching sick patient care. If you count immunizations, screenings, and checkups, there is some sick patient *prevention* care but very little natural wellness. There is a growing trend to move to a wellness modality, including preventive medicine and healthful lifestyle training. Healthcare costs and disability costs are some of the most worrisome parts of the federal budgetary troubles. These costs can be greatly reduced by healthful lifestyles. Will this happen before the economy and an individual's bank accounts go bust?

Easy Takeaways

1. Once you see millions of years of history that show how humans once moved, you fully understand how the modern era has been

robbed of one of the most natural of human activities.

2. Unlike some hibernators, most branches of the animal kingdom (humans have long been listed as part of this) lack built-in mechanisms that can keep them healthy and well without physical movement.

3. A growing trend is a prevailing avoidance of activities that produce huffing and puffing, increased circulation, and endorphin-type highs. Lack of physical movement directly equates to unnatural living and the breakdown of mind and body.

4. Evolution has programmed us to hold onto calories, storing them as fat, for long winters or other periods of food scarcity.

5. Although I say the 1970s equal sedentism, physically unfit citizens were a problem much earlier on. Exercising's history goes way back. In 1956, during Eisenhower's presidency, the President's Council on Physical Fitness was organized as a response to unfit American children (as compared to European children).

6. In the modern era, the 1970s mark a big line in the sand for the downward spiral of socioeconomic trends in the West. Sociologist Ira Goldstein points out that the early 1970s ring in the beginning of the decline in U.S. standard of living largely based in a decline in domestic productivity.

7. Experts and regular citizens alike are rallying for a societal move to a wellness modality, including preventive medicine and healthful lifestyle training.

Chapter 4
Survival Guide for the Sedentary World

The only exercise some people get is jumping
to conclusions, running down their friends, sidestepping
responsibility, and pushing their luck!
—Author unknown

Freedom: taking a step outside of a temporary conformity to fix broken patterns and flawed comfort zones. The liberation starts with the first step. Freedom is not license to do whatever you want. True freedom is doing the right thing naturally. Maturity is when we are doing more right things.

circular reasoning: if there ever was a paradox, it's a person who claims to be too busy for physical activity and other wellness pursuits but has plenty of time for eating and drinking unhealthful stuff between meals. This type of reasoning causes damage to our sit bones (aka sitz bones) and fills in that area with bigger circles so that the person now has their own built-in butt pillows. Another oddity is the would-be health-intentioned person who says the fitness, yoga, or martial arts center (or group, class, or personal trainer) is too steep a monthly cost (at perhaps $150) but then spends money on pricey Botox shots, elective cosmetic dental work, and "health foods" like synthesized supplements and red wine.

less is more: You're bogged down by work, home, and other responsibilities. But if you say you are always too busy to do the right thing—for instance, taking care of yourself—you are not being intellectually honest.

Let's imagine for a moment you're in a small hotel suite on a budget vacation. I know from experience how happy many people are when spending time away from home in a small hotel suite. Your office knows only to call you in an emergency. You have time to visit the tourist office and plan some excursions as well as time to do nothing (though rest and downtime are not nothing; they're part of nature's laws for healthful living). You have easy choices in apparel because you choose from the select few outfits that fit inside your carry-on suitcase. You may prepare one or two meals a day right at the kitchenette and then dine out. You're happy.

How goes the wellness practice of physical movement when you're in a hotel, have plenty of time to recreate, and are away from your stuff? If you still blow off doing a complete exercise program and avoid physical recreation, then you have your answer. You are suffering from the lamentable condition of wellness avoidance. That means you aren't taking care of yourself.

If you want to finish a mentally taxing project or bond with your significant other, get away from your stuff by checking into a hotel. Or clean out your home's finished garage, and pretend …

success: it's a journey, not a destination. The shortest distance between two points is …? a straight line

"I've been working all my life to become an overnight success."
—Author unknown

our current status: we are either in a state of prepare or repair. Contemporary wellness theorists would probably agree that given our current health crisis, as a stressed out society, we are in a state of repair.

control: manage your decisions well everyday. Learn to control yourself and not expect too much. In general, goals should be realistically attainable except perhaps in the cases where we are called upon to be a superhuman: Joan of Arc, Sampson, Mighty Mouse …

organizations: In general, the underlying motivation of most any organization is to sustain itself. Directors are normally hired and rewarded for their ability to keep the organization thriving. Some have been hired because of their ability to win, no matter the means. "Whatever it takes …"

Recruits Welcome Speech

"Recruits, my job over the following weeks of basic training in wellness is to ingrain in your minds, and in your hearts, that movement is a normal and necessary part of everyday life.

1. It should be functional
2. And it should be recreational.

"If you are not open to being convinced of the benefits of movement, get out of line and back on the couch. Unless you are ready, willing, and able to move, my coaching won't help you do anything besides waste time."

That is my MacArthur/Patton wellness speech. Both were young officers during the First World War and were asked to train soldiers and staffers over the courses of their illustrious careers. This speech stems from my belief that we tend to overanalyze and babble about the vagaries of daily life. Better we get to the doing. Go through the daily list and get things done. If you want help in preventing the need for a hip replacement, keep reading.

In an overwhelming majority of cases, these are the primary reasons Westerners have stopped doing physical activities that provide fitness:

As we grew older we adopted a completely different lifestyle than when we were young. Today, this is a tricky subject since so many of our youth are sedentary from the start.

Physical activities are no longer part of recreation—a pleasant pastime; they've become challenging work, just like our day jobs.

Knowing this, the answers to the problem of lack of fitness are obvious:

1. Never grow up completely and never stop playing.

2. Never stop recreating.

Instead of choosing the simple, direct route, many grown-up people have a propensity towards excessive analyzing of data and options. With so much daily time spent considering and perhaps belaboring options, they wind up not doing what they actually know is right and natural. This guilt drives binge eating and time wasting. These people may yak with friends in lengthy venting conversations where nothing much gets accomplished.

People know how to avoid sagging bodies, nagging pain, and anxious minds. They know that binging is bad and that intentional body movement provides physical and emotional release. But they tend not to do it. The default setting is yesterday's pattern of inactivity and binging. What do you think about resetting the default to invigoration, sex appeal, and euphoria?

> **Question:** Why do kids generally occupy themselves with nonstop play at playgrounds?

> **Answer:** It's fun and natural for them to have energy and use it.

Why do most adults sit or stand around these days when their kids are playing? Are their kids so at risk and needy they require spotters and kidnap prevention at every turn? Unfortunately, because of the potential risks these days, some parents and policy-makers will answer yes to the kidnap prevention question. Once kids reach a point of self-awareness, can parents do their own exercise program while their kids are enjoying self-directed free play? Can parents still be watchfully present while engaging in their own fitness movements? (See Operation BITWIC on the Net for my answers on this.)

Well, according to this new survey, three out of five parents say ...

STOP with the surveys! These ubiquitous info-blasts have become absurd. Stop, I say. Instead, use your bodies and minds and make some wise choices that will benefit both.

Did You See the Latest ... ?

Tuning in for the constant deluge, we adults demonstrate powerlessness in controlling our hunger for more news. Don't forget we are modeling this behavior and our anxiety to our kids. Because of the pervasive and invasive nature of sound, noise, and stress, we impart some of this news mania to our kids who, instead of discovering and enjoying much of their own play, are spending way too much time on electronic devices. Endlessly watching Internet pop and prank videos, keeps kids following the lives of others and is taking time away from more beneficial activities.*

We adults are no different. Our frequent impulsive choices act like plunging anchors to our development and wellbeing. In this way, our development suffers periods of retrograde or stagnation. If some of this is comprised of sedentism, gluttony, and the worry that accompanies the first two, our everyday choices wind up creating havoc for our bodies and dispositions. The answer to our problems and voids, it would seem, is only one digital click, download, or self-help article away. If it's not, why are we forever reaching for "the latest" instead of using our common sense and intuition? The common sense approach should, one hopes, lead to living as a natural human being who consumes high-grade fuel, engages in daily movement opportunities, and enjoys life. And this natural human being would have

---

* Beneficial activities seem so obvious. But to many, they're obviously not so. Ask an artistically inclined fit friend what they think about this subject. I can't imagine they will tell you that watching after-school TV specials is as enjoyable or as engaging as playing an instrument or roller skating.

the good sense to turn off the electrical gadgets, enjoy downtime, and connect with others in family time and social settings.

Whether we're clicking online or listening to on-air updates, endless articles and news briefs filter through our visual and auditory horizons every day. We get blasted by the news. Psychologists call this "information overload." Author Richard Louv says that we are doing more and more indoors (and I add, *in cars*) and this trend is increasing. This reveals how we may be suffering from what Louv calls the "nature-deficit disorder." When we get out in nature and observe things and lose ourselves in its mystery, Louv says, "You are immersed in something with all our senses that you don't know you're paying attention. You lose awareness of how immersed you are. That is the best antidote to the burnout that technology in particular creates for us."

Some additional benefits of getting out in nature:[20]

1. Nature, including the color green, generally lowers stress and our heart rate.
2. The fewer the buildings and man-made things, the more we connect to nature.
3. Fresh air fills our lungs. The more we move, the more we take in and expel.
4. We make vitamin D from the sun.
5. We appreciate the natural relationship of the flora and fauna.
6. We see things close up and at a distance. Viewing these differences is helpful for our vision as well as our brain chemistry.
7. We can bond with others in a natural setting.

Better Than Overanalyzing, Get Up and Get Out and Produce Vitamin D

Whether or not you experience an enlightened, Zen-like state, nature still provides benefits to your conscious and unconscious mind. It supplies both health and freedom. Remaining indoors, especially for endless periods of time, tends to equate to confinement and sedentism.

Unless we live in a green house, those indoor periods are certainly not providing any vitamin D. The only popular vegetables that contain vitamin D are mushrooms—interestingly, it's one of the veggies that doesn't require much, or in some cases any, sunlight. Unless you are sucking down mackerel fat or broiling salmon, you are probably not getting the vitamin D you need. For this and many other reasons, the outdoors is where you should spend some time. As you do, you will produce one of the most important of vitamins.

There are studies galore that tell us how to live. Some of us read them, then email the more incendiary blurbs to our friends and spend time in conversation at the dinner table on the subject of the newfound knowledge.

Some studies are quite helpful since they contribute fresh information that compels us to do things in a better way, or even drop deleterious practices completely. For example, somewhere along the way some policy body or research institute thought it might be a good idea to get arsenic out of households.[21] Once upon a time every local cop and generalist physician in the Western world knew that arsenic was too accessible and people were dying from ingesting it, some by error—such as young children—while others came to greet the big sleep because their spouse started sprinkling it into their morning coffee ... a variation of "breakfast in bed, dear" ... (a *dirt* bed alas).

Other studies exist partly because they give scientists something to do. You'd have to admit, with huge numbers of doctoral students graduating each year, including a good number whose career paths land them in scientific research—a profession whose ranks have swelled into perhaps the tens of millions—not all of their studies are going to be of pivotal import. How many of them are going to be attempts at providing us with more natural lifestyles achieved with peaceful happiness and durable integrity?*

A significant and growing number of these studies are going to be outright sponsored studies, initiated by a company desiring to sell a product or technology based on the study. Plenty of technical job candidates will be snapped up by the defense industry, including a number who work on building better weapons and technologies for killing humans and destroying nature, water supplies, and a country's infrastructure. This, of course, can't be coming as a surprise to you.

Picture the scene at the 20-year high school reunion in some town in America (or Ireland, which in the new millennium, put together a leading high-tech defense industry). "Did you hear about Sandy? He was a lead engineer who invented some of the technology used to bomb Iraq. His devices blew their sewer systems to smithereens."

---

* Beryl Lieff Benderly's February 20, 2010 article in Scientific American says, "According to Harvard professor Richard Freeman, there is no shortage of scientific labor. 30,000 scientists and engineers—about 18,000 of them American citizens—earn PhDs in the U.S. each year."

"Wow," comes the reply followed by another sip of the reunion punch. "Well, he always was good in science."*

Fixalls

Can't we simply stop buying into the myriad of the latest in pills, potions, and fixalls? As far as health and wellness are concerned, learning how to live a natural, balanced life is without a doubt more vital than reading the plethora of latest articles. I would wager these articles and online reports are being read while people are sitting down. Not that I'm against reading well-intentioned guideposts, but if our main problem is lack of active movement, how much time should we be spending seated, reading about the subject? Moderation is the key.

Having authored this book, I would hope that periodically reading about the subject of movement may provide a chance to learn a new mindset that could help us all improve. But make sure you don't get excessively addicted to reading the latest stuff. Believe me, I do a bit of that and it can eat away at your time and peace of mind. If you get too involved with this you may find yourself without time to handle the other necessities of life. It was explained to me that the total of information on health and wellness currently doubles every four years. This suggests that it's humanly unfeasible to attempt to take on a significant percentage of that.

It's easier to let someone else digest the latest studies. If you

---

* I am not here to categorically bash scientists, doctors, and other highly educated people. The wielded club is squarely aimed to do a bit of system bashing. The system pays scientists and doctors to work a certain way to enhance the wealth of the controllers of the system, not always to improve the lives of the masses who live under the system.

find a trusted "digester" of information, you can read their updates and see what they say. Then crosscheck that information and opinion with another source—even one who may disagree. There are a number of well-intentioned wellness blogs available. Find the ones with the least ties to big corporations. As you are able, read a few wellness books and articles on occasion. Look for the authors with the least ties to the material world's systems of untruths. The ones preaching natural approaches make the most sense to me. If the expert is someone who works intense, 15-hour days and doesn't have time to take care of themselves or their loved ones, that discounts them in the book of natural approaches.

As always, perhaps the best use of your time on wellness is to use your intuition. You know that your body doesn't respond positively to soda, donuts, and being seated all day. If you can't stop gravitating to these products and practices, your intuition should share that you are an addict who needs help. Take yourself in to see someone who can help. If you are already in a good place without too much in the way of negative practices, just keep enhancing your practice of wellness. Keep moving and keep pondering. In fact, ponder while moving and do both frequently. Forget that—work this process into *every* day! Start the day with movement and pondering. Once you get into the groove with this practice, centering yourself should happen quite naturally.

In the pages of this book, I have done my utmost to, as they say, "tell my audience something they don't already know." Perhaps the composition and condensing of cultural shifts of the Timeline has done that for some of you. Maybe you'll find some newness in a philosophy that steps away from the machines of mega-gyms and pages of research studies as it embraces some of the thinking and daily movement patterns of our ancestors, both family farmers and hunter-gatherers.

How do I know about what they were thinking and how they were moving?

Because I lived it.

Important Wellness Action Step— The Hunter-Gatherer Lifestyle

Much of my mindset is based on the wisest of the hunter-gatherers: wake up and move, hunt and gather, rest and heal, release and ponder, care for and give thanks, commune with nature and others, sing and dance like everybody's watching, and tread softly and live. I say "wisest" because hunter-gatherers were not always sufficiently skilled in their planning. Throughout history, untold tribes overpopulated areas, destroyed habitat, and waged war just as we do.

Growing Up in the Country

Good fortune allowed our family to live on a small farm that was surrounded by the larger farms. In the 1970s, my family had the opportunity to visit farms, some of them generations old, on a regular basis.

My father excelled at teaching us new things. As a regular pattern, he had us review what we had previously learned. Much of this occurred on car trips or while working in our fields and garden. He taught us how to ask questions, how to be a good listener, and how to keep a conversation going, often with the use of openness and humor.

Together, we struck up conversations with farmers, gardeners, and others with specific knowledge (and interesting life stories) wherever we traveled. In the 1970s, there were no pure hunter-gatherers where I grew up—though I did grow up hunting and fishing, and I still eat wild berries.* Hunter-gatherers still inhabit our world today. Carefully considering their lifestyles as I read through books and watch documentary films has produced an understanding where we (and they) seem to have gone wrong. To sum it up in one sentence: We are consumers who can never get enough; they tend to live in the midst of nature and learn things from it. Doesn't survival depend on harmonious living? Reading up on the disappearance of cultures—like the Rapanui of Easter Island—helps put this question in perspective.

Information on hunter-gatherers, including the Native North Americans, is readily available, and it's just as important to know about their social history, as it is to know about the world's political history that we are typically force-fed in school. I hold with those who argue that social history, learning how ordinary people lived, is far more essential in a person's education. Life should be more about just living it rather than tuning in and being bombarded by a bunch of central government hullabaloo ... as long as tanks aren't rolling down our streets ...

Even if the tanks are positioned nearby, we still need to acquire food and have something to do. Knowing how to work with the land and sea provides food as well as productive activities. Would you rather flip channels than go on a boat ride? If you answered

---

* A frugal and adaptive man once told me that he gathers, takes home, and eats fruit that falls off trees located near the sides of roads. He calls this "road fall," a play on the term "road kill."

yes, then a conversation with your great-grandmother may be warranted. Séance, prayer, reading her poems or letters, or simply allowing her to talk to you might be the ticket.

Where Else Should We Look For Answers?

Some of the best health knowledge might easily be acquired by connecting with our best friend as well as by communing with our ancestors.

A Dog's Life

Who lives more naturally and is more removed from the age of TMI (too much information)—people or dogs?

What would our dogs say if they could talk?

"Allow me to run and roam. That's what my four legs have done since even before we were dogs. Our ancestors, the wolves, used our appendages to track and hunt, and still do. Today, I'd be happy with a walk in the morning, one in the evening, and a doggy door to a shady spot in the backyard or balcony.

"And another thing—I can talk. That's what I'm saying when I drag the leash over to you and go berserk when it's high time we headed out. When we get to the park, do you mind if I roll around, jump over things, and chase anything worth chasing? I really like to be silly and love it when you turn off your cell phone and get your silly on too!

"And remember when you were in grade school and high school and you used to watch us running around *off leash* and often wished you could be running with us? I know, I know, you played sports all year round, but you still envied what we were doing, right?

"And one more thing. You monitor my chow so that I don't become overweight. And I've gotten pretty used to eating the portions you feed me. How 'bout you let me decide what type and how much chow you get so that you maintain your desired weight and stop expelling so much gas around the house? I'm glad you don't feed me soda because my teeth are most helpful in eating, gnawing toys, and guarding our communal area.

"Woof, woof, sure, sure, exercise and eating right takes some work. But these practices are far less challenging than a colonoscopy. I'm only going to be around for 10 to 15 human years. You may be around for a few score more than that—increasing your chances of bowel disorders. You can start your new program by not sitting around so much and eating never ending portions of sugary, greasy, and mushy foods."

The Moral of the Story

When daily activity and diet monitoring is handled by a caring, no-nonsense coach (with big canines), it has a high rate of success.

Workbook Moment

Ask yourself: if you were a counselor or coach and you walked in, what would you tell you to do? (If you own this book, write your answer here. If you have the digital version, jot these down separately.)

1. _____

2. _____

3. _____

So, why aren't you doing it?

Great-Great-Grandma Weighs In

What would great-great-grandma say if she could still talk to us? If you have aged family members around, ask them to share their wisdom.

"Chores had to be done. I got up before dawn to get things going in the house. My husband was already out checking the animals before that. He'd come in with some fresh milk and eggs, and I'd prepare a nice breakfast for the whole family. Working the land, we survived by knowing things. One of those things was to keep moving all day. Even if you folks today are strapped down on your butt most of the time, you've still got to get your blood flowing somehow. You've got to look deep inside and figure it out. And no complaining, y'hear?"

Disregarding the wisdom of grandma is a dereliction of duty.

You might check in with your ancestors. Don't think, "pick up the phone." Go outside and take a walk and think about them. Think about how they made it through their harsher situations. Consider the mindset needed to survive long days of physical labor, raise oodles of kids during times of scarcity, and overcome other life trials.

A few of my ancestors long gone still provide me wisdom, motivation, and help in times of crisis. All it takes is a bit of time and trust to allow their words to fill you up with goodness and resolve. There has to be a good egg somewhere in your lineage. If you are religious, talk to God. If you are spiritual, talk to the great spirits. If you are a lover of history, talk to someone like Ben Franklin. If you are like me, talk to all of the above. In times of greatest need, I talk to my grandmother who passed away shortly after I graduated from college. She was one of the most helpful and humble good eggs in my family's recent lineage.

The Moral of the Story

Complaints don't hold up in the court of grandma.

"We are what we repeatedly do. Excellence, then,
is not an act but a habit."
—Aristotle, who developed a science of happiness
(384 B.C. – 322 B.C. Ancient Greece)

If work, meals, and commute take up 12 hours per day, should we be hitting the gym for another hour or two? Some of the more prominent motivational public speakers have been advising us all to get in a few hours of learning per day—reading, taking classes, plotting our course, seeking counsel, and so on. And let's not forget communing with family. I continue to remind people to get family time. The authors of books on long-lived cultures cite how those groups known for health and vitality typically share living space with family and typically share at least some meals with extended family. This lifestyle is presented as a principal, common thread to all cultures rich in centenarians.

"Is there a connection between respecting elders and longevity?" asks author Dan Buettner in his 2012 book "Bluezones." "Absolutely," he has found, and the good tidings are shared by all in the family. "Seniors who live at home are more likely to get better care and remain engaged," he writes.

Buettner notes how the seniors he spent time with in Sardinian villages contribute to the household chores and provide a living legacy of wisdom and level mindedness. This helps both the seniors and the younger generations who live near them. For the seniors,

Buettner shares, "They have strong self-esteem and a clear purpose. They love, and they are loved."[22]

Setting and embracing such priorities is pivotal in our personal, familial, and communal wellness.

When I explain mindset and mind over matter to people in our modern era, I often say, "Can you imagine the force of mind that old-school farmers in Nebraska [which seems more bucolic than my native New Jersey] had to have when using a scythe to cut large plantings of grasses and grains? The only way they could have done that is by tapping into the realm of mind over matter."

Can you imagine the invigoration, the exhaustion, and fulfillment you might feel when you were done with that? Your bone structure, musculature, and mind would have you feeling almost superhuman!

Post-physical activity, we experience feelings that are often spectacular. The science can break this down in a myriad of positive responses from our physiology and brain chemistry. Even our genes seem to receive a boost. Some studies have found that one part of the exercise payoff provides wellness at the genetic level. Increasing research has been studying the rise and fall of telomeres that cap the endings of human chromosomes. Longer telomeres are present in thriving, healthful individuals. An article in The Journal of Aging Research mentions that "longer telomeres are associated with higher physical activity levels, indicating a potential mechanistic link between physical activity, reduced age-related disease risk, and longevity."[23]

Reading these studies in detail, you learn that more exercise is not always better. The stressors present in extreme endurance athletes can wind up shortening telomeres and causing other severe problems, including fatigued athlete myopathic syndrome (FAMS which is a chronic fatigue brought on by overtraining and is considered irreversible), musculoskeletal problems, and organ dysfunction, not to mention family breakup. Besides the genetic problems and other biological problems (see free radicals and renal problems) extreme endurance athletes often endure these setbacks:

1. Traveling too frequently.
2. Focus on training, diet, and rest overtakes most other activities.
3. Too tired to be available for other members of family.
4. Frequently injured.
5. Have a difficult time balancing work, training, recovery, travel, and family.

One caveat to mention is that we can all get excessive in anything we do, whether it's work, tennis, or even spiritual endeavors. Yes, we can even O.D. on church and spiritual studies and meetings. Even if we're not OCD, we may plunge in to our next program of activity and disregard the advice of others who tell us "we're pushing too hard."

In whatever we do, it's important to keep up a framework of balance. In physical activity, pain and excessive fatigue are often good indications of when we're overdoing things. Having done distance running for more than three decades, I've learned what my body appreciates and doesn't appreciate. I've always been attuned to the idea of pacing myself. I don't keep going when my feet are killing me. What would be the gain in that? When I get to the hereafter, I'll remember to ask Pheidippides, "Why was it so important to bring news of a Greek victory over the Persians?" If you recall the legend, he pushed himself so hard in running from Marathon to Athens that he dropped dead after delivering the news.

Wellness is not about pushing yourself to more distant finish lines. It's about listening to the wellness call of the body and the mind. If you aren't yet a runner, start your trek by walking and hiking. You'll know when there's ample spring in your step and drive in your heart. If you listen closely to the body, not the ego, you'll know when to pick up the pace or go an extra mile. In the next section, you'll be reminded that excessive or improper sitting can cause breakdown just as cataclysmic as overtraining.

No Complaining

That's a tall order for many of us in the sedentary world. Many are tired, achy, have indigestion, and experience memory lapses. An article I came across today was featured on page D4 of a copy of the Wall Street Journal. Found in the Health & Wellness section, it was entitled "Years of Sitting on the Job Linked to Cancer." The article cites a study published in the American Journal of Epidemiology that links sedentism not only with chronic conditions such as heart disease but also with colon cancer.

How do we utilize our energy while sitting? Our brains use lots of energy but that doesn't create the same healthful response as physical activity. Activities are considered physically sedentary (what this book shortens to the term *sedentary*) if they require very low exertion. The obvious example is prolonged sitting. In a previous study, subjects who spent 10 or more years in sedentary jobs had twice the risk of colon cancer and 44 percent increased risk of rectal cancer, compared with those who never held a sedentary job. Occupations requiring heavy activity were associated with a 44 percent reduced risk of colon cancer compared with light-activity work.[24]

News like this hits us right where we sit! Did you really need any study to tell you that? If you did, where did you misplace your intuition?

Rather than causing endless worry, emphasis on *end*, articles like these are a wake-up call. The point is to steer clear of our tendency to overanalyze, and instead get moving. The less we grumble and the more we get our bodies doing some meaningful, appropriate moving, the less tired and achy we are, and the more the body is happy and in balance with the mind. This means taking up what's known as the holistic approach. This means not pigeonholing ourselves by concentrating on just a few aspects of a healthful life, but living life with a wide angle of good practices that make us happy and well and of good service to all. The more we work with our system and maintain balance, the less our system creates cancer cells and other problems. It really is that simple.

If you get that and live by it, you can read the rest of this book for what I hope you will find artful muckraking; workable wellness tips; some modern East-West philosophy; and some real-world tales you may find motivational, educational, and entertaining.

The sum of blame for sedentary lifestyles should not land on the backside of the common person who was born into it. Every crime has its usual suspects. In the case of sedentism, we could name the Protestant work ethic and the current sedentary job offerings. We could also name corporate control of policy as well as Homo sapiens' innate tendency to be poor planners. Evolutionary survival training may have us programmed to minimize energy expenditure. Beyond that, there's always good old progress. Electricity and the TV worked well together to promote sedentism, obesity, and unwellness. And poor diets played right into the promotion—feeding junk to the immobile, inactive human machine. The following is a potentially helpful way of rendering the story of sedentism.

The Five Branches of Sedentism

Branch One: Villages

Communal sedentism, fixed villages with domestication of plants and animals, was a choice the ancients began developing about 12,000 years ago.

Branch Two: Disconnection from Nature

The second branch is overpopulation and disconnection from the land and sea, where all of our food and most of our visual and earthly happiness comes from. To be clear, overpopulation of portions of the Earth was evidenced long before communal villages. This was how some ecosystems were wiped out and wound up killing off populations.

Branch Three: Too Much Time in Static Positions

Then there's the deplorable third branch of sedentism—sitting in chairs, benches, and the like for long periods. Standing for long periods also engenders psycho-anatomical dilemmas. Active movement also means changing positions frequently and resting as needed. Sitting properly and comfortably in meditative, yoga positions—or squatting down comfortably as cultures do around the world—directly benefits human biomechanics.

As mentioned in this book's historical Timeline, ancient schooling, as utilized during the Roman Empire to train soldiers, was one of the early examples of obliging large groups of people to sit, often on the ground, or stand idly for relatively lengthy periods. Evolutionary researchers suggest the adoption of sedentism is a natural human tendency toward energy conservation. Starting this in the home and at school also indoctrinates young people with the proposition that sitting is a way of life.

Sitting eventually became *the* way to get smart and eventually get a career. The cross-section of Christian churches initially had worshippers standing during service before pews were installed. History reveals a practice of not moving for most of the duration of typical church services. Even today at any speaking event, remaining virtually motionless during the lecture is often considered the proper thing to do. Through the Common Era, it became more prevalent for houses of worship to require sitting. Though this was for much shorter periods than educational and vocational institutions would come to demand. Some of the most non-sedentary Christian services I've been invited to attend were the Catholic masses that had us transferring weight between sitting, standing, kneeling, and then rounding the pews for host and wine. Gospel churches are also reputed for their share of moving to the groove.

Be sure to watch the acrobatic service in the original Blues Brothers' film. Has the spirit ever moved you into flight?

Sitting isn't always a stationary pursuit. Sitting as one grinds wheat or maize into flour isn't the same as sitting to follow a school lesson. Which is more physical? Which provides more rump and body movement?

What can the discerning, humble, and lighthearted mind draw from all of this?

You need to sit for hours or all day if you want to get smart or weave a rug. But a religious experience only requires sitting for an hour.

Branch Four: Disability

The fourth branch of sedentism occurs when you are partially or completely disabled. Here you are bedridden or confined to a few different table-like and chair-like apparatuses. Bedsores and rashes are all but unavoidable. Typically, reaching this branch diminishes chances of returning to customary human physical movement.

Branch Five: The Eternal Rest

The fifth branch is what American detective fiction-writing icon Raymond Chandler—and the Mafia hit men who adopted his term—called *the big sleep*. Once your body arrives in that drawer, the mausoleum's steel door closes and the mind may finally relax since it is no longer preoccupied with life's worries. In today's terms, you're no longer wired to and from digital devices. The body can get all the rest and peace it needs.*

---

* Old customs die slowly. We should, however, let some of these customs die. Thinking organically, some choose to bury the physical remains (of the person who has left their body) in the ground in an organic box. This may contaminate the ground and potentially the water table. The astute tribal people burned their dead, not breathing in the smoke. We can cremate human remains and spread the ashes on a special place and quit spending so much time, energy, and money on the preservation of dead cells. We don't need hundreds of millions of casketized remains and our families don't need to spend $100,000 honoring, burying, and storing the bodies of our four grandparents. We can honor their spirits without fixating on their bodies. Honor the marker, the tombstone, or the urn. To teach future generations what we were up to, we can save some bodies, but not the majority. Is it kinder to a dead body to slow down its decomposition?

Easy Takeaways

1. It's understandable that we are sedentary—we've been programmed to sit and listen since childhood.

2. Though a box has been formed, we have to think outside of that box.

3. Long ago the Greeks pioneered gymnasiums, and gyms are effective for some things. But, to make a change in your fitness level, you don't have to "get back to the gym." The closest safe outdoor space will do just fine. If you need to use the greater indoors, do so.

4. We live in a world of TMI (too much information). At regular intervals, turn it all off and get to know yourself. Tap into your own innate intelligence and internal force.

5. Sitting or standing for long periods does damage. Excessive physical effort harms us. Step into the realm of balance.

Chapter 5

Recreation and Physical Activity

Movement, recreation, and downtime are big parts of the message I preach. The modern problem lies less in not knowing what exercises to do than in not moving much at all. Yes, consuming healthful food is immensely important, but food is fuel for movement and human functionality, not an uncontrollable and frequent antidote for boredom or depression.

Let's examine a small part of my own family and contacts' history of movement via a photographic record. This section may help prove "The answers to many of our wellness answers are not found in the new millennium; they're found in 1910."

Photo Section

2010 testing 1910:
The moveable parts still worked 100 years later.

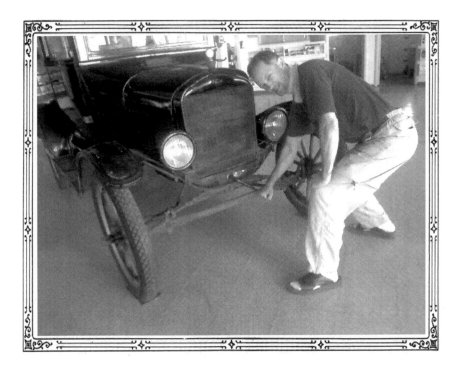

Old-school living demanded plenty of physical activity.

There were no mouse clicks or home-based remote controls. Your grandparents or great-grandparents did lots of walking. When the automobile became popular, many of the West's ancestors still continued walking. If an average family had a car, there was only one per household. For many there were the basic chores of mopping, chopping wood, butchering a goose, hauling water, and tending the garden.

Back in the old days, even automobile users had to have the strength and technique to fire up the engine.

Everyone should use proper posture—a long-backed ectomorph like me, Sifu Slim, simply must. Without the posture and technique, I'd throw my back out. Trust me, I've done it repeatedly.

This book, and my philosophy, is not about extreme living or transformational weight loss; it's about doing the right things and enjoying a life without gluttonous addictions.

Some of the call to movement presented in Sedentary Nation may seem a bit challenging for some. Well, carry this with you: I'm not asking you to do something I haven't already done.

If a twig like me—a five-decades-old guy who has spent most of his life sitting at a desk and now a computer—can do decline push-ups, chin-ups gripping a martial arts belt, jiu-jitsu with 20-year-olds, and lift a 50-pound bag of salt out of the car …

Kenoga Lake, Mass., 1910. One of the most straightforward of field and lawn games—wheelbarrow races.

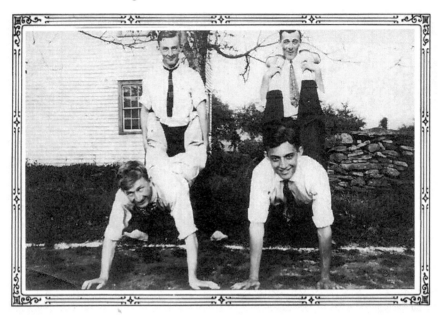

When I was little—in the 1960s and '70s—we couldn't wait to test our agility through games and skill activities. Frequently we hear of new-millennium kids who don't want to be "bugged" with requests of doing "physical stuff."

My maternal grandfather, Louis II, second-generation German-American (all of his grandparents were of German ancestry), is shown here, bottom right, with a group of his friends. Louis graduated in the 1912 class of Barringer High School, Newark, New Jersey. Founded in 1838, it was the first high school in New Jersey and the third oldest in the United States.

A cross-country runner, he had the same build as me. I have ectomorph (thin stature) grandparents on three of the four sides.

Who do you think generally wins the wheelbarrow races? The skinny and long, the short and squat, or the behemoths? After a good warm-up, try it and see. Then consider the concept of core strength.

Some of the answers to our physical and mental wellness are found in the same year as this photo: 1910.

What do you think they are?

Kenoga Lake, Mass., 1910.
Being Silly and Letting off Steam ... Outdoors!

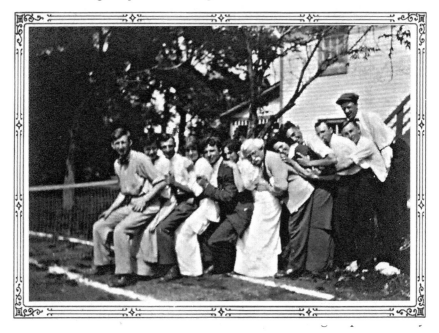

skinny folks enjoying life outdoors.

Note the mustachioed Mark Twain look-alike.

Louis II is fourth in from the right. These people weren't doing body boot camp or transformational workouts. They just ate less (especially junk carbs), snacked less in general, and consumed less bagged food like chips. They walked frequently, and got outside to recreate. My grandfather was especially fond of peanuts which he spent time peeling from their shells. At times during his generation, the larger meal of roasted meat was often a special meal reserved for Sunday afternoons.

No one (except perhaps the industry capos themselves) is saying to eat more factory-farmed, steroid- and antibiotic-laced protein and fat from meat, but we need to eat more healthful fat. This argument leads us back to the myth of foods with naturally occurring (considered healthful) fats creating heart problems. Dissenters to what's known as the diet-heart myth say that saturated fats and cholesterol are not the problem. Eat some healthful fat—avocados, seeds, nuts, fish, eggs, and, if it sits well with your system and your path, the best meat you can afford. Didn't you know that low-fat diets have come under severe criticism lately? Here is what a good number of the experts are now agreeing on:

- The pancreas produces insulin, which is one way to produce body fat, and simple carbs signal to the pancreas to spike insulin production.
- The following foods contain excessive amounts of simple carbs and should be avoided: soda, pizza, beer, pasta, cereal, cake, and candy.
- Some nutritionists include potatoes as banes; some do not.
- Avoid diets higher in carbs and any foods containing sugar and corn syrup.
- Avoid eating sugar, which releases several hormones—including ghrelin, the hunger hormone. This can create even more hunger. Healthful proteins and fats satiate the stomach and the brain. And so do nutrient-dense vegetables.

Why do some food-industry critics believe food marketers produce food with reduced fat and 0 percent fat?

Because of profit of course. No fat is perhaps the biggest food gimmick of the past half-century. Food marketers are playing into our ignorance about the cause of weight gain. By consuming low or little fat, we eat more of the products, especially when they're laced with sugar or corn syrup. The number one thing that has to change if we are going to get well is the sedentary nature of our brains.

Asbury Park, New Jersey Shore, 1914.
Recreation Without Digital Gadgets

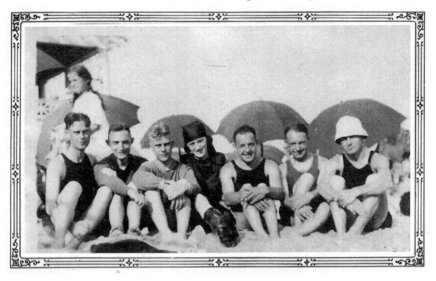

Louis Rissland II, second from the left, with his crew of "recreators."

True, there were some sedentary folks in the pre-World War II days, but to most folks, a day on the beach meant a chance to play: riding waves, swimming, walking, tossing balls, chewing saltwater taffy, and even—if you can fathom it—being silly. Occasionally a game of cards would break out, and frequently, a cigarette would find a flame. But most people weren't sitting idly downing bags of crapola waiting for a phone call or text.

How many hefty people do you see in this photo? Do you know how regular people become supersized?

They typically do it a few pounds per year. That's known as "creeping obesity." Two pounds per year over 30 years equals 60 pounds. What does four pounds per year equal?

Olympic Park, Irvington, N.J., 1922. Recreation

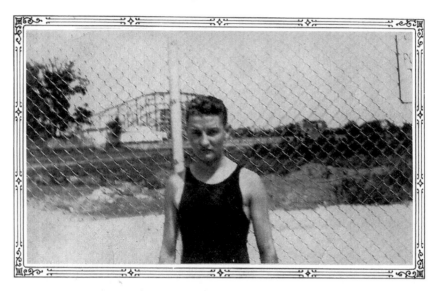

My paternal grandfather, Henry Kreuter II, b. 1904, is shown shortly after his graduation from high school. They called him "The Prince" because he was the youngest of five kids; the others were his elder sisters. Despite working five-and-a-half days a week during the Great Depression while raising a family, he usually found some time to walk through a weekly round on the golf course.

One thing I like to remind is that fleshy people did not make up the majority in previous generations. Most people were active and thin, especially during their youth. And yes, diet did play a part. Calorie consumption has gone way up since the times of my grandparents. Today's generation consumes as many as 400 to 1000 calories per day more than their great-grandparents. And lots of it is comprised of highly processed food and simple carbohydrates: sugar.

Of course, in prior eras, there were people of varied bone structures, musculature, and body-fat percentages. But the record shows only a small percentage of "beefy" young people a generation or two ago. Look at students in college these days. Compare their physiques to people in college in the 1940s. Look at the photos of the men and women joining the effort in World War II. Even before they went in to train, most of them were slender. Though many were not fit.

Flesh-wise, my thin physique is quite similar to the young soldiers entering and exiting boot camp in World War II. Even after five decades of a lot of sitting, it's a blessing that atrophy still hasn't set in. Physical movement as a daily ritual (plus stretches or walking during the day) has prevented that. The physical movement program I call The Maintenance Workout connects mind, body, and spirit. It incorporates focus, smiles, laughter, and attitude adjustment all in one.

Spring Lake Beach, New Jersey Shore, 1979. Surfing Cousins

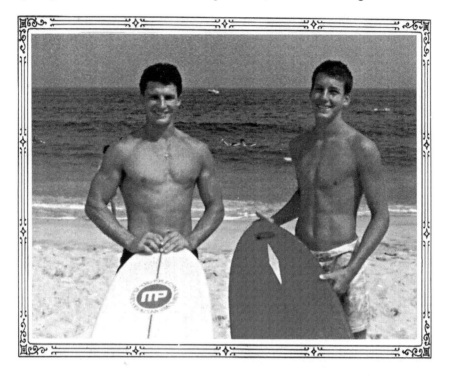

My cousins, grandsons of Henry II. Henry Meehan, b. 1959 a competitive fitness legend, and his brother, David, b. 1963. Henry is a former Marine and winner of a long line of police and fire fighter strength and endurance competitions.

Henry and I have been talking about doing talk radio, sort of a fitness and wellness reality-check version of the hilarious "Car Talk" show with the self-deprecating Tappet Brothers from Boston.

Henry does a training program that includes tire flipping. Some of the tires he flips, end over end, are so humongous, most people would think they're immovable. David, also an accomplished athlete, put on 35 pounds of beef since this photo with his own steady fitness program. Had he been a vegan, he might have put on 35 pounds of chiseled tofu. They both have raised kids, toiled long hours, endeavored to be good husbands, and still found time daily to "get physical" and get a daily release.

Maplewood, N.J., 1938. What almost looks like a scene out of the musical "Oklahoma" is actually the New York City suburbs.

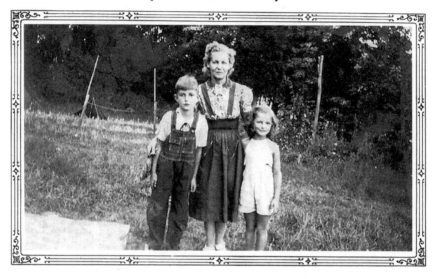

We often forget how recently sprawling suburbia came about in the United States. Here my father, Henry III, grandmother Nell, and Aunt Cookie bring a rural look to the suburban landscape in the Garden State. My first hometown, Maplewood, is 25 miles east of Manhattan. The featured WWII generation and my own 1960s–'70s generation were known for mothers who kicked their kids out of the house after breakfast and chores saying, "Go out and play."

They did the same thing after lunch and after dinner. If the weather demanded it, galoshes and parkas meant the rule was still the same: "Go outside and play with the other kids." Moments like those give parents some time for whatever they need to do—including quiet downtime and intimacy.

Cape Cod, Mass., 1968. Family Day at the Beach

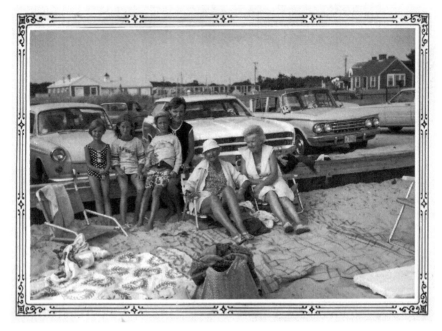

My sisters, Gee and Heidi (in New York Rangers jersey); me; my mother, Ruth; Mrs. P., a family friend; and my maternal grandmother, Georgina Rissland—the only medium build of my grandparents.

Family, friends, and neighbors of all generations are meant to spend time together. This is how wisdom gets passed down and fun interaction happens naturally. Keeping up with fit and agile kids is a natural, recreational way to stay active.

Did you know that the recent stats show arguably the highest percentage of people living alone in the history of our species?

Does digital social media remove burdens and enhance connection, or does it create excessive disconnection from rubbing elbows with our fellow humans?

Lake Champlain, N.Y., 1977. This was as fun as it looks.

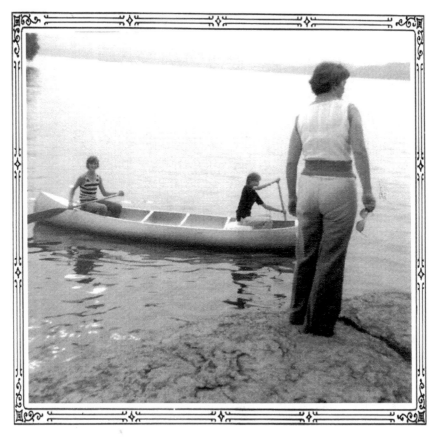

I steer, my younger sister, Gee, paddles as my mother, Ruth, surveys the action.

Would you agree that recreation is a heck of a lot more fulfilling than texting and video games? We kids never worried about dropping our smartphones or MP3 players into the water—they didn't exist. We didn't carry any electronics on our person, so we were not getting zapped as much by electromagnetic frequencies as modern, new-millennium kids.

We had fun swamping canoes and then righting them to paddle onward. You don't see shorts in this photo, but we kids became much more adapted to water when style and sense had us swapping out our cut-off jeans for nylon beach shorts. Jeans shorts took forever to dry out. We evolved and accepted some of the modern advancements. Clammy garments are no fun.

Tewksbury, N.J., 1977. Animal Husbandry

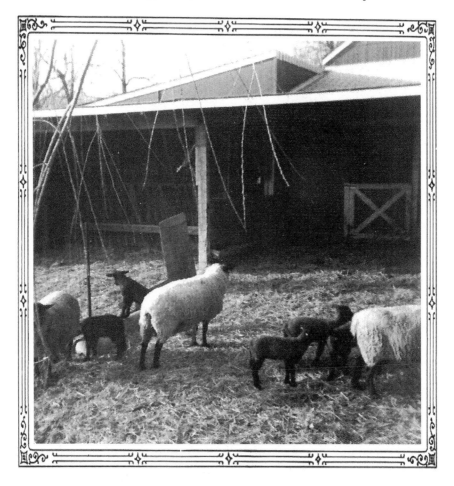

We moved to rural New Jersey in 1972 when my parents decided to buy a farm. We were always amazed how the sheep had their own built-in barometers. The ewes frequently gave birth to their lambs right during a snowfall. Here, in early spring, the lambs are four to six weeks old.

Involvement in the 4-H Sheep Club had us kids learning many skills at an early age. Among those were animal husbandry and public speaking. We thought it loads of fun to attend the meetings and eat delicious country potluck than always be hanging around the house, farm, and neighborhood.

Change and movement are some of the keys to an engaging life. You never saw Grizzly Adams playing solitaire on his computer. Would a modern remake of the 1970's TV series have a cabin with a satellite dish and solar cells?

Christmas 1980. Time for Arts and Crafts

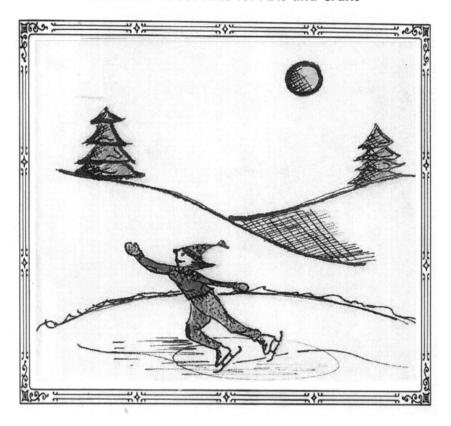

A Christmas card made by my sister, Heidi. This mirrored what we kids were doing in the frequently cold and dreary New Jersey winter. Even in the rain, we were outside each and every day. Can you picture the artwork that would mirror what many kids are doing these days? Would it have kids on the floor playing digital war games or animated sports games on the big screen TV?

The farm, almost 40 years of rural living for my folks. No sheep anymore, now it's Christmas trees. My mother, Ruth, shoveling snow.

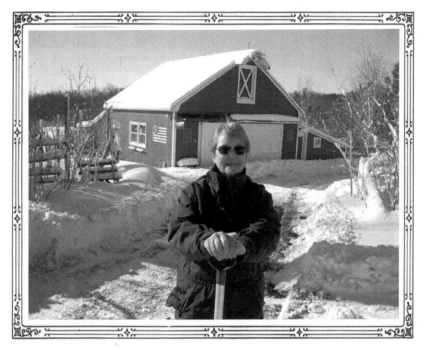

My parents' part- or full-time job—depending on the season— had long been taking care of their land and buildings. By doing so, they were able to gain physical activity, fresh produce from the large garden (behind the snow pile on the left), and camaraderie from the merry visitors to Wyndemere Farm who come and watch as their chosen tree is cut fresh for their holiday enjoyment.

My mother, Ruth, had been doing water aerobics for several years. But rather than being a gym person, she more easily gravitated to farm and housework—physical exertion with a dual purpose.

New Millennium. Tewksbury, N.J.
From Wall Street to Snow Drifts

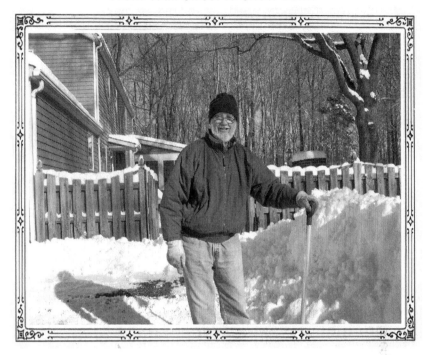

My father, Henry III, worked as a journalist for two different Olympics as a young man. Then he spent 30 years as an institutional stockbroker before retiring from 2 World Trade Center in 1989.

He loves to get out of the house. Here, in mid-winter, he enjoys the sun and fills up on vitamin D as well as Schumann resonances (look this up).

Many of my friends snickered when my father had aluminum siding installed in the mid-'70s. This 1960's Colonial still has the same wood shingle siding it was built with—under the aluminum. The aluminum still looks good almost 40 years later... so does the able-minded man who made that wise decision.

West Sacramento, Calif., 2002. A Decompression Work Out

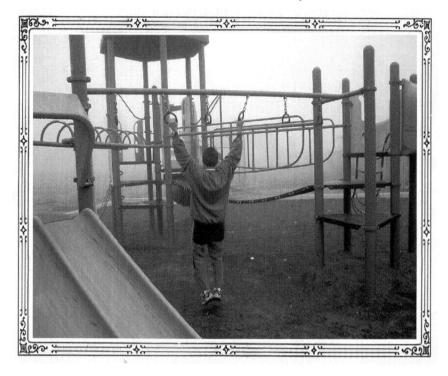

To pay bills while pursuing the passion of writing, I worked for several years doing plumbing and home remodel work. Struggling artists (and corporate people out of a job) normally have some kind of hourly work going to keep afloat.

My friend, Fred, demonstrates chin-ups using kids' play area devices. He was so strong with bodyweight exercises that we wound up strapping weighted SCUBA belts on his waist. A former lumberjack, elite fitness practitioner, and cyclist, Fred, came over from Aix-en-Provence, France, to work construction and train with me for a time. We hit the kids' playground for Marine-style "bar workouts" at 6 a.m. in the foggy winter and showed up at the jobsites to demo floors and run new pipe a few hours later. He suggested we take days off on the weekends. I was paying back my costs from living for half the year in Europe and told him, "When there's work these days, we work."

Sometimes I was able to convince him to don his construction attire on Sundays. Yes, I have had many months and semesters devoid of what I think is critical to human wellness: downtime. We sometimes do make sacrifices to stay afloat in the material world.

Would you agree that if we fed ourselves properly and intentionally moved our bodies daily that we'd be setting a course towards wellness?

What do you think of the idea of spending some time in physical activity in fresh air, with nice people? And being silly?

2002, West Sacramento, Calif. Workout in the Fog

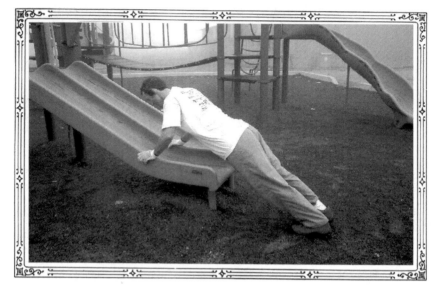

Me exercising while listening to my Sony headset radio. Yes, I'm getting zapped in my brain by radio waves and electromagnetic frequencies, but an invigorating outdoor workout helps negate some of the damage of indoor, sedentary living. Now I usually do these workouts barefoot to be electrically grounded to the Earth.

I'm outside five to seven mornings per week, usually in the same dozen or so workout areas. The music or radio programs I listen to help keep things from getting monotonous. There's one beach in Santa Barbara where I've worked out and run a circuit loop so frequently, even the seagulls have gotten to know me. What are they telling me when they dive-bomb my van? Who knows, but so far they have yet to dive-bomb my headset radio ... or my head.

I hope to see outdoor exercise areas for adults—search my program "Operation Bitwic" (build it and they will come, from "Field of Dreams") on the Net. But, until that time, I and many others use whatever we can to get in a full-body workout.

Here I'm wearing hospital scrubs and grippy gloves while doing incline push-ups, part of the exercise circuit I do which has helped minimize my chances of needing to go in for surgery ... and last rites. Do you think it makes any sense to eat junk and drink sugary drinks after expending time and energy every morning on fitness, wellness, and connection to nature? None whatsoever. If you get up and start the day with a coffee and a donut, it's easy to maintain a lackluster, junk-filled existence. By the same token, if you eat well, it's easier to keep clean with the rest of your wellness routine.

Hit the blog at *SedentaryNation.com* with your thoughts.

South Carolina, 2009. Not much time spent in mid-life crisis for this *bad hombre*.

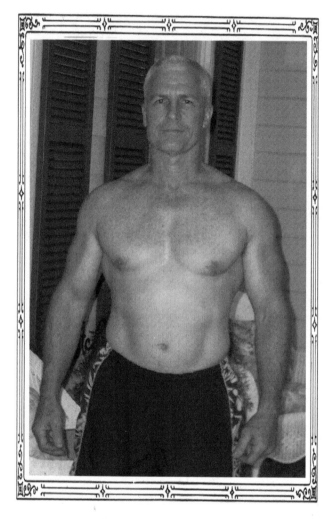

My cousin Henry from the New Jersey Shore, here at age 50. This former lieutenant in the Marine Corps is medium build (mesomorph). He trains, competes, flips tires, fishes, surfs in stormy seas, and presses people's buttons—especially when he thinks them less than reasonable. Henry also leads prayer groups and Bible studies. Even the Good Book mentions warriors. Since this one has a sense of humor, I told him to write a book about his high-impact workouts called "I Never Met a Tire I Didn't Like."

I show my sweetheart his hair color and tell her, "This cousin is three years older. Plan for it now. What hair I still have is going to look this color." I've been trying to get Henry into jiu-jitsu, aka the gentle art. He has been trying to get me to flip tires. Eventually, one day I did find myself taking up tire flipping.

Quebec, 2009. Massage Envy

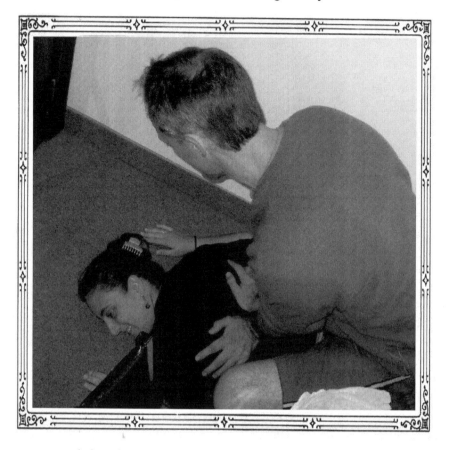

I travel the planet passing on what health and healing assistance I can. Here, right in our classroom in Canada, I take a moment to perform Shiatsu massage on a young physician from Central America. When we were done with that, the good doctor was feeling well enough to do some salsa dancing with me. I don't get how people go from one sedentary class or work-team meeting to the next and are able to keep their mind, body, and spirit together. Recess should be for all ages, not only for young kids. The job-site break room just ain't cuttin' it.

Santa Barbara, Calif., 2008. A Long Flight from Dublin

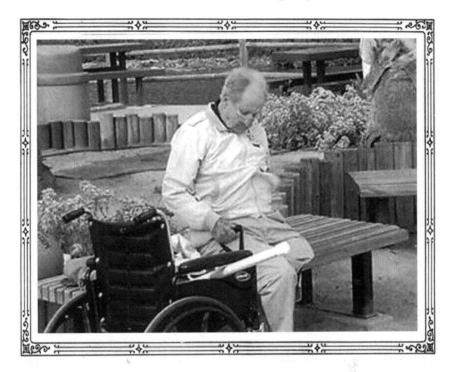

This 94-year-old retiree, originally based in New York, told me he was considered too old to enlist when WWII came around. For nearly his entire adult life, his only fitness plan was walking the distance to and from work. Then, in his 80s, sitting for 12 hours on a long flight from Dublin to California caused DVT, deep veined thrombosis (a blood clot in a deep vein in the leg), and an emergency landing.

Emergency surgery removed his left leg. From that point on, he became a slightly older version of Jack LaLanne. He told me part of his life story and how he had been "exercising from this seated position several hours per day for over a decade. This is what keeps me going."

In his hand is an elastic resistance belt he has anchored by his right foot.

What keeps you going?

Will it take a major health incident to provide motivation?

Surfers Point, Ventura, Calif., 2006. Life is about balance.

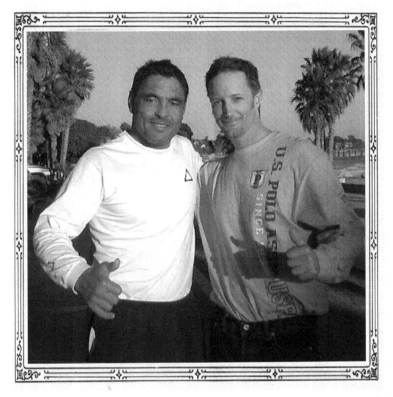

The modern version of Bruce Lee. Rickson Gracie, an eighth-degree black belt and known as "the purest example of the Gracie family's Brazilian jiu-jitsu," is an avid surfer. Approaching the end of his fifth decade of physical, mental, and emotional feats and challenges, he makes time to connect with nature and ride early morning waves—what I call "a free ride from God."

When sharks see this guy's sleek, honed muscles, they swim the other way. Hopefully, not my way. When I asked this grandmaster for some life wisdom, he paused for a moment then said, "The secret of life is to be silly. No, forget that. The secret to life is to be silly all of the time."

Christmas 2011. Taking Rickson Gracie up on his recommendation of being silly.

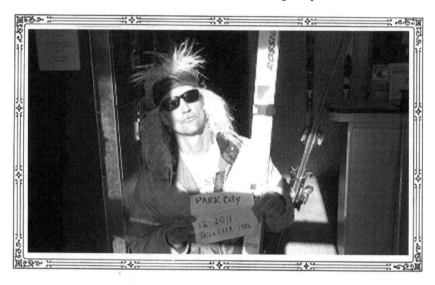

The guys who resurfaced my skis in Santa Barbara told me to ditch the old 1980's skis.

I told them, "They were good then, why couldn't they be fine two decades later?" When I picked up this 1980's jump-suit at a yard sale, I knew I had to give the whole ensemble a try. The David Lee Roth hair, well ... let's just say I like costume parties. See more of this breaking trip down Big Hair '80s Lane on YouTube. Search "Sifu Slim 1980's skis."

Santa Barbara, Calif., 2009. Speaking Engagement

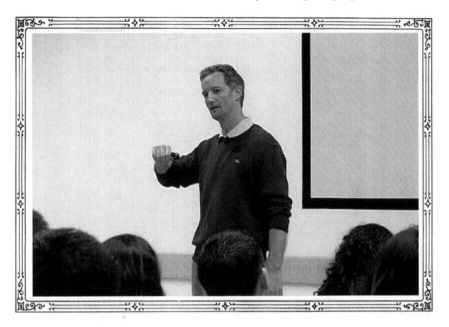

I'm speaking about wellness in front of a group of engineering students who are seated or in bed nearly 95 percent of their average 24-hour period. A number of these folks—aged early 20s—complained of ailments related to their sedentary lifestyle.

Don't hesitate to dial the Sifu Slim hotline if you want me to pack my bags and come deliver a well researched and easily implemented wellness message with some fun and tension-lightening audience involvement. So far I can deliver it in English, French, or Spanish—or to keep people awake, in all three.

Q: "How does the new millennium chicken get across the road?"

A: "On his own mobility scooter."

The modern-day factory-farmed chicken is so pumped up on steroids and so obese he can't walk. Guess who eats him? So much for animal husbandry in the hyper-productive world.

1970 Pittsburgh, Pa.

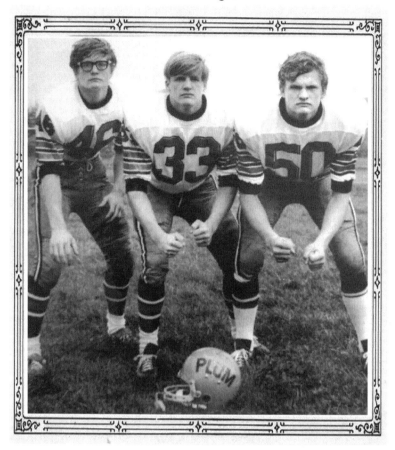

My next book, "The Aging Athlete," asks the question: "Why do most competitive athletes and former military personnel wind up in a frequently sedentary lifestyle of pizza, beer, desks, and couches shortly after retiring from competition and service?"

A group of elite fitness, endurance, and skill athletes weigh in. So do some former elite athletes who are now couch potatoes.

Here in the standard, old-school eyewear is my second interviewed athlete. Grandson of a coal miner, son of a truck driver, Pittsburgh native Mac McCluskey played a larger man's sport. He told me, "My older and much stronger brother (no. 50) used to kick my butt!" His cousin, no. 33, doesn't look like a small dude either.

Mac wound up playing college football at Arizona State and semi-pro football in Pittsburgh. His drive for accomplishment is amazing.

Clermont, Fla., 2006. From Team Sports to Triathlons

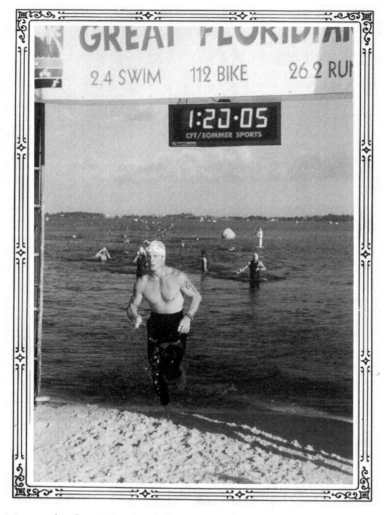

Now in his late 50s, third-degree Black Belt in Tae Kwon Do and triathlete since the early days of the sport, Mac lives in Park City, Utah, where he still trains every day and coaches other elite athletes.

One of the highlights of his life came during a period when he was depressed. A horrible auto accident had left him disfigured and unable to compete in his action-packed sports like football and baseball. After reconstructive surgeries, he left the East and sought his fortune and a new life in California, where he was picked up by a fellow citizen as he hitchhiked in Los Angeles. The gregarious man who drove him to his destination told him, "Never give up. You have something you want, so go out and get it. I have faith in you."

As the 26-year-old Mac closed the car door and said his farewell, he looked at the driver and noticed it was none other than the godfather of fitness and motivation, Jack LaLanne.

For more info, see *TheAgingAthlete.com*

To send someone a digital or print copy of this book, go to *SedentaryNation.com*

Easy Takeaways

1. Euphoria is wonderful. The fact we seek to experience it is normal, desirable, and part of our human reward center—just like what parents feel when their child steps into another moment of miracles.

2. Adequate rest, as is repeated throughout this book, is a big part of proper metabolism (including calorie burning) and wellness.

3. Instead of thinking, "you are what you eat," think, "you are how you live."

4. One way suggested to reduce EMF exposure is to place plants around the house—big and rangy house plants like spider plants, rubber trees, and palms which are said to absorb EMF waves.

5. Before going to sleep, cover all of your light sources, or do what I do and wear a cozy, fleece sleeping beanie that can be pulled down over the eyes.

6. The photo section takeaways. Spend some time in physical activity, in fresh air, with good friends. And be silly.

Chapter 6

Movement and the Hunter-Gatherers

Anthropology: the study of ancient and modern human cultures with the intention of learning about them and, hopefully, from them.

imagination: You use it or lose it. Just like when taking in the radio story hours of yesteryear, listen in and create your own images.

Here's the Question

How did (and do) the hunter-gatherers move?

Upright-walking non-apes are suggested to have started as scavenger-gatherers and moved on to hunting and gathering. If we include them, we're talking about a history of perhaps at least 6 million years of upright walkers, so just considering 19th-century tribal peoples—say in Africa or New Zealand—doesn't paint very much of the historic picture. Though, it certainly is a good way to start. If that's not enough, older folks and film buffs will recall Raquel Welch in "One Million Years B.C."

Can you picture a cave dweller? A jungle gatherer? A Nordic hunter? A tribe of Mohawks in North America?

Think about how they lived. What images come to mind?

The images I've come across in my mind, in books, and film say they sometimes crawled to sneak up on prey. They ran for safety, to attack, and to persistence hunt. Persistence hunting is what a group of fit hunters can do in the heat of the day. Since animals can't cool off while they're running, hunters run at them from different angles, keeping them running long enough until the animal overheats, stops, stands there or collapses, and ultimately surrenders. We know some even ran for the fun of it, aka diversion. For more on this see the book "Born to Run."

Hunter-gatherers climbed, stealthily snuck, and held anatomically challenging positions. They stooped over; hoisted heavy objects on their backs, shoulders, and heads; they worked while kneeling, sitting, and squatting. Their feet were active and their jaws did lots of tightening and clenching while working. Their hands—both sexes—were strong and able. All of this biomechanical strength and endurance spelled survival.

Ever wonder why old movies and literature talk about "marrying a strong woman or man"? No one wanted to wind up with a disabled partner or one who might die in childbirth. People wanted to live a full, active life and sought to have their progeny survive.

Once you're in shape, try some of this. If you want to emulate some of their movement patterns, pretend you're Tarzan running, climbing, swinging, or swimming to save animals and Jane. Imitate

Jane climbing across river rocks and swinging on strong branches. Go around objects: trees, posts, road signs, and cones, whatever. Practice your full-body dexterity: Climb around on bars and jungle gyms. Crawl on all fours, not on your knees. Do jiu-jitsu or wrestling. Play ultimate Frisbee or lacrosse. Vestiges of lacrosse were found in Mesoamerica and Canada, dating back to the 17th century. If you're old, achy, or unfit, make sure to get fit and take care of your weaknesses before starting a strenuous program.

Seekers of an easy parking-lot or sidewalk game with demands of physicality and balance might take up hopscotch. Why did we ever stop playing that wonderful game of coordination and one-legged vigor? If we kept it up, hip and knee replacements would go way down—and so would early death.

Aren't we supposed to gain intelligence with age? Then why do we move from games with biomechanical brilliance and little chance of injury to one-sided or one directional activities that often lead to biomechanical breakdown.

Tennis and golf are wonderful games, but they are up there on the list of sports that cause joint injury—and for many, aggravation. One of the biggest gripes about golf is the frequent slowness of play. Hopscotch increases dexterity and functional strength. It is not a one-sided game of more forceful starts and stops—like tennis. Nor is it a one-directional, harsh, impact sport—like golf. Golf and tennis are wonderful for recreation and getting outdoors, but they require functional fitness. It's not advised to go out and smack balls when you have structural weaknesses and pain. Or when you are not warmed up.

To build up and trim down, play Jacks in a sweat sauna. No, forget that. Just play Jacks getting up every five minutes to do some crazy dancing or some Bernie Lean. Google this to watch a simple new millennium dance form you may decide to try—your body willing and able of course.

Lifestyles of the Functionally Famous

Millions of years of existence have programmed us to seek active ways to move our human chemistry around. The idea is to keep it circulating, taking in good fuel, keeping the motor and chassis free of debris, and allowing it to rest and cool down as needed. We were also programmed to rest, or celebrate and commune, when the food acquisition and other chores have been accomplished.

Parts of the definition of "rest":

1. a bodily state characterized by minimal functional and metabolic activities
2. free from anxiety or disturbance[25]

To assess the following statement one should first consider the big picture of millions of years of human existence and then compare those lifestyles with other communal creatures that live off the land. Hunter-gatherers are the best example of humans who moved around and generally got plenty of downtime. When the food supply was ample and efficiently accessible, their workloads and survival stresses were reduced.

If they had to work long days to attain the needed calories and nutrients or if they had to spend lots of energy on keeping warm or safe, the duration of downtime was substantially compromised. One could argue we don't actually know what they did. I don't think it's that difficult to imagine.

Humans (and animals) enjoy a variety of activities. Some things were taken up communally—like chanting, eating the bigger meals, and banging on beats on drums. Some past-times might have been taken up solo—like wandering or pondering. When a tribe's basic needs had been provided, it's not too hard to imagine moments of playfulness, entertainment, forward planning, education, and rest.

Some bands of hunter-gatherers still exist and can be seen enjoying lots of downtime hours. See the Hadza in north-central Tanzania, and the Pila Nguru (aka Spinifex) in Western Australia. Starting in the 1990s, the San people—aka Bushmen or Basawra—were forcibly removed from their native lands in Botswana's Kalahari Game Reserve. To do this they had to become farmers. Read into their ongoing plight, which is reported to have to do with the billion-dollar diamond and mineral mining potential held in their ancestral land. It should be noted that numbers of San had already moved to farming and herding in the mid-20th century.

What about animals and downtime? Prides of lions experience life with a significant potential for downtime. Downtime is how they roll. When they obtain their food on the hunt and scavenge, lions then have time for other things. The same thing goes for hunter-gatherers. Successful and fortunate hunter-gatherers were not and are not working long days plowing fields, harvesting crops, and delivering baby animals which would be routine, intense responsibilities that scads of farmers undertake.

Our farmer ancestors worked long and hard days. Farmers still work hard today. Remember why slavery came about. It is sometimes easier and more economically viable to house workers and force them to work than remunerate them fairly to do it. Consider a contemporary commercial farm that hires seasonal workers. During harvest season, workers are regularly paid by the pound or basket of what they have picked. The pace at which these pickers work is almost unfathomable and not generally conducive to an enjoyable day. For the individual, this backbreaking work is not generally sustainable over the course of years.

If you have ever planted a garden, set tile, installed new landscaping with drainage and rock walls, or built an addition on your home, you know how hard that type of work is. Now add in having lots of kids and taking care of them. In the U.S., seven kids was the average in the year 1800, a time at which most people lived in rural areas. 3.5 was the average in 1900 for people across the United States, in both urban and rural areas.[26]

Now move to the urban centers in the late 1800s and early 1900s. Our ancestors did lots of walking and most worked with their hands. Scores who worked in industry toiled away in relatively fixed or extremely fixed work stations where they would perform repetitive tasks: assembly lines, clothing manufacturing, food processing, and dock labor. Many of these jobs created injuries for workers. In general, injured workers were immediately replaced by others who, in some cases, had been hoping someone would get sick or hurt so that they could land a job and help feed their families.

The building of the Golden Gate Bridge (1933–1937) took place during the Great Depression. Destitute, unemployed men reportedly waited and watched the employed workers, hoping someone might get injured or fall to their death. Due to safety netting, the death wait would mostly prove unsuccessful. The construction resulted in a safety record of only 11 deaths, though plenty of ironworkers got sick from the burning bolts. During the installation process of metal beams, metal bolts were heated up red hot. This produced a toxic smoke that caused workers to get sick and lose their hair. When these ironworkers became ill, the waiting unemployed got their chance at a job.

Proper Physicality at Work

This scale considers the *general picture* to rank the physicality of 19th- through 21st-century Western job lifestyles based on customary practices. Exceptions are standard. The role of this table is to provide a starting point for discussion. It is a general and not comprehensive look at the subject. It is, however, based on careful consideration using experiential knowledge, interviews and anecdotal evidence, and reading. This is not a scientific study. Do we really need another study to prove that repetitive stress, endless sitting, and harsh activities are harmful?

Ranking For Proper Anatomic Physicality and Peaceful Downtime (1 to 10 Scale)

Hunting and gathering: (Before modern era, thus without modern encroachments. Sans constant war. When protein and fat are readily available.) — 10

(With encroachment from modern world. With low protein and fat sources. You are effectively working too hard for your food. Though this mandates constant cooperation, which can provide a tribal plus.) — 7

Old-school, small-plot farming: (Better scenario: small farming that is seasonal. Shared work. Canning food seasonally. Some hunting and fishing to provide recreation and food. Winter with more downtime.) — 8

(Worse scenario: little downtime, little cooperation, working oneself to the bone.) — 6

Grand-scale, modern farming: (Too much mechanization and sitting. For the lowly individual: constant stress of debt, the corporations own your soul, and market forces create constant uncertainty. You may take a vacation but it's not a sure thing. You live knowing what you are doing is detrimental to nature.) — 6

Physical workers: (Field labor or people—including contractors, gardeners, etc.—who work until exhaustion and rarely get time off. The 5–8 ranking depends on the abuse vs. health this provides.) — 5–8

(Skilled and "unskilled" laborers and those who use their muscles most of the day and work steadily, generally choosing not to keep going until exhaustion: contractors, gardeners, massage therapists, mechanics, lifters/loaders/movers, etc. Many suffer repetitive stress injuries.) — 6

(Chiropractors, physical therapists, P.E. teachers/athletic coaches, personal trainers. Lots of movement, very little sitting.) — 8

Confining industrial work: (Lots of working in fixed positions and repetitive stress; assembly lines—like manufacturing and factory meat processing; people as machines.) — 5

Service economy: (An active Desk Potato who does things right and exercises. In this case there is generally too much sitting in chairs.) — 6

(Sedentary desk potatoes, car/truck potatoes who engage in little or no physical movement at work. This person practices little or no fitness and does not pause for periodic stretch brakes. Downtime is often spent continuing the digital overload.)   4

(An active delivery person like a UPS driver who is fit. UPS has been known for their decent pay and great benefits. That has to positively affect their demeanor and team ethic. Active and retired firefighters I have talked to mention the high number of their fellow workers who retire early with disabilities. This makes it difficult to rank them. On the one hand you have the fit or at least functional; on the other you have relatively young people who are permanently/partially disabled.)   8

(Better scenario: Some move more and do some bending and lifting, i.e., a convenience store person who sweeps, lifts, stocks shelves, and cleans.)   6

(Worse scenario: Little movement. Movement is generally one sided and repetitive: a tollbooth operator who sits, turns, and leans the same way ... and breathes fumes.)   3–5

Why do some of these categories rank lower than industrial work? It's really a toss-up. How can you pick the more detrimental path out of a number of lousy situations? Here's an attempt. Some movement, even if it's repetitive, might be considered better than no movement, for example, "It's better to wear away than to rust away." That's not to say that creating dysfunction is a good practice.

Contemplating daily life and work activities via a gross overview fitness and wellness analysis—full range of motion, getting the heart rate up, using a natural posture, getting plenty of downtime, eating fresh, native food, etc.—the hunter-gatherers are the group to assume generally enjoyed better health than other societies. Fossil records show many examples of strong bones and teeth—as well as some periods of malnutrition. Anthropologists have found endless evidence of bone fractures, especially in the feet. There is also substantial evidence of worn-out teeth.

Neanderthal skeletons in particular reveal high incidence of fractures. One conclusion is they frequently hunted large animals with spears, which suggests trauma experienced in almost a kill or be killed environment. At the very least, it seems to present a kill or starve environment. Another take on this is the more you are physical, the more chances you have of hurting yourself. Obviously, Neanderthals had higher chances of trauma injuries than desk potatoes. Talking to baggage handlers at airports has helped me realize how challenging it is to prevent injuries when doing endless physical work. Even greater risks are faced when we become a human part of conveyor belt machines. Repetitive stress and hurried handling create chances for injury.

Those who have made studies of extant tribal people conclude their heart health and anatomical structure health is generally exceptional. A report published in "Hypertension," the journal of the American Heart Association, praises the heart health of tribal people who live off the land.

Coincidentally, the other two groups mentioned in the report also have a close relation with food. In fact, their movement patterns are mostly related to food acquisition. Says researcher Dr. Michael Gurven, "Age-related increases in blood pressure have been observed in almost every population, except among hunter-gatherers, farmers, and pastoralists who have traditional lives and grow only what they need for survival."[27]

Important Note: Moves to Modern Lifestyles Are Easily Traceable to Wellness Woes

Take the Inuit, aka Eskimos. The first offspring raised eating Western diets experienced high incidence of myopia. One study by ophthalmologist Elizabeth Cass concluded, "Before the year 1940 among the Inuit people (of all age groups) in one region of Canada's Northwest Territories, myopia was non-existent." When the Inuit children were moved to boarding schools in 1940, within "a few years time 100 percent of the relocated students became myopic. Cass attributed this form of rapid ocular degeneration primarily to adverse changes in their nutrition." Processed foods have been cited as a main cause.[28]

Most would agree we can't go back now to being hunter-gatherers. But there are movements afoot attempting to develop closer connections to food. The buy local and buy organic movements are attempts to promote the viability of responsibly grown, nourishing, fresh food. Numbers of city and town dwellers (including yours truly who has had expansive gardens in the past and has also grown food plants in large pots) are currently trying their luck with aspects of urban homesteading—planting food gardens and raising small livestock in residential areas (urban and suburban). Also look up the *slow food* movement.

What can we do to emulate the natural movement of the hunter-gatherers?

In terms of a practice of natural movement, one way is to look at combining the techniques of some active movers we are familiar with. I talk a lot about combining the movement programs of Bruce Lee with Jack LaLanne. Both were talented in strength and balance. Both had great tempo to their movements. Calisthenics was Jack's forte though he also used machines and swam frequently. Bruce was known for trying everything in fitness conditioning. His speed and grace in movement were remarkable.

To those two programs, we mix in some limited-sole (aka thin-soled) running. The big mistake people often make with running is the over emphasis of running for weight loss and health transformation, rather than maintenance and euphoria. Too many also tend to concentrate on running's drudgery or endurance. Don't forget the sprints, hills, intervals, and crossover steps. Playfulness is a wonderful part of running. Drudgery is a drag. For a fit and healthy runner, playful running may be rewarding and fun. For a person who is not in sync, running rarely moves into the realm of euphoria.

I like to mix in some hiking, swimming, and some crawling on hands and feet. This morning's multi-directional five-minute program of crawling was no piece of cake. On a summer's day, recovering from a hot night and less-than-optimal sleep, I had to get my will up to do it. This was a day after explaining to my aged father how to maintain bone density and muscle tissue through the aging process. I told him to use leg power and good posture to get out of a chair with no hands. "Do that 20 times and see how you feel."

Pushing 52, but still 31 years younger than my father, I had to "man up" and take care of myself. So, I did five cartwheels and then began to crawl. Putting weight on your body in that position is extremely beneficial, and, it's an incredible workout.

Jack LaLanne always pushed himself. It was as though he were competing with himself, trying to surpass his formerly younger self. Among other things, Jack LaLanne spent time testing and honing his body and mind with surf paddling—on his stomach. Just holding your shoulders and head up on the board for paddling is an incredibly taxing. For those long in the back, it can be exhausting. I speak from experience.

All good intentions aside, practicing lifelong movement activities these days is oft considered quite challenging. For most of us, we won't do long-term physical movement unless (a) we have time and energy, and (b) it creates a joyful release. To enjoy it most and make it last for a lifetime, do it all with a joyous, light-hearted attitude. If you're already doing that, you know the magic that provides.

"A mind that is stretched by new experiences
can never go back to its old dimensions."
—Oliver Wendell Holmes, American Supreme Court Justice
(Boston 1841 – Washington, D.C., 1935)

I would add these words to Holmes' quote: open and accepting. Thus, "An open and accepting mind that is stretched by new experiences can never go back to its old dimensions." That way, the quote helps us better understand those who relapse.

Addiction could be defined this way: Continuing to do something detrimental no matter the consequences. People who use almost all possible means and are still unable to break addictions may have but one last step—lockdown.

If they aren't locked down, severe food addicts open the fridge in the same way a drug addict opens an unlocked window—of someone else's house.

Taking an accounting of the typical modern family, most would contend that old patterns are hard to break, especially when they deal with gluttony, addiction to digital devices, unhealthful eating, and inactivity.[29]

Jack Lalanne, the Godfather of Fitness, Was a Sugar Addict

Jack LaLanne—a sick kid and sugar addict—wasn't on his own. In 1929, when the world was on the cusp of a financial nosedive, young Jack started his personal move to wellness with the love of his parents and then some heartfelt counsel handed down by nutrition crusader, Paul Bragg. This spark happened all in one day and night when Jack's mother took him to hear Paul Bragg speak. "My mother and I sat in front of 3,000 people," Jack recalled. "It had to be the most embarrassing, and humiliating time of my life. I didn't want anyone to see me, and I thought they were all looking at sickly me. Little did I know that most of them had health problems too!"[30]

I'll summarize a bit more of Jack's life.

He was one of the smallest kids in his neighborhood in Berkeley, California. Jack was sickly, weak, had boils and pimples, and wore a back brace. At age 15, suffering from bulimia and depression, he dropped out of school and remained mostly inside his parents' home. (Don't forget that vitamin D deficiency can worsen depression.) He was afraid to show himself in public.

He met Paul Bragg, American self-made guru of natural diet and healthful lifestyle, while Bragg was on tour in California. After speaking at length with the guru at the event center, Jack was helped to see the light. He went on to become a graduate of chiropractic school, receive the title of the "godfather of fitness," start the first chain of physical culture gyms, star in the longest running one-person TV show (1951–1985), publish 10 books, complete a number of amazing feats of fitness, and create personal wealth, especially from his juicing machines.

I believe his biggest asset was attitude—he never gave up on himself or the masses. Never a star who was too busy to stop and share a laugh and some wisdom with Jane and Joe Public, Jack was always a positive guy.

Here is a quote that shows how driven he was. In his blog entry, Michael d'Estries writes, "He had an attitude described as fierce, but even Jack would tell it straight if asked. When questioned whether age ever got in the way of his goals, LaLanne once said:

"I train like I'm training for the Olympics or for a Mr. America contest, the way I've always trained my whole life. You see, life is a battlefield. Life is survival of the fittest. How many healthy people do you know? How many happy people do you know? Think about it. People work at dying, they don't work at living. My workout is my obligation to life. It's my tranquilizer. It's part of the way I tell the truth—and telling the truth is what's kept me going all these years."[31]

Two things to remember about him:

1. He exercised every day, which he said was never easy.

2. He never gave up on people.

So Jack found some answers when he got to meet Paul Bragg after the speaker's talk. That same night the adolescent LaLanne prayed. He put a stop to his addictions by ridding his diet of sweets and took up the wellness lifestyle. Now, a scholar-athlete, he would fill his day with positive activities and go on to become a world class fitness athlete. In his 20s, Jack completed his degree in chiropractics. His depression vanished and he got well. After a time, he taught others, got married, began a family, and eventually had millions of viewers and listeners. He was rarely alone.

He was not alone even when he exercised by training in the individual sport of swimming. Not only did he often have other swimmers swimming beside him in lanes, but also, during his millions of breast strokes through the water, he was in the company of himself: pushing himself from the outside—Jack the coach; and pushing himself from the inside—Jack the student. Though he spent lots of quality time with other people, including his wife, Elaine, Jack did a lot of self-coaching.

Former karate world champion Bob Wall traveled with Jack LaLanne on a promotional tour for six months in the mid 1970s. I asked Bob about Jack's workouts. "He worked out right in his hotel room. He brought along an apparatus he'd put over the door for chin-ups and leg raises. He'd do push-ups and sit-ups and all kinds of calisthenics. He didn't need a gym."

"Did you give it a try?" I asked.

"Jack knew his abilities in fitness were beyond the elite level. He could do repetitions a gymnast would have trouble with. He had a standing bet which he offered me. 'If you can do my entire workout, I'll give you $10,000.' My answer was, 'Okay, as long as you'll take me up on my offer, $20,000 if you can beat me in physical combat.' Besides buying each other some drinks, no wager winnings ever changed hands but I did work out with him on occasion."

Jack was not alone; hunter-gatherers were not alone, the lone wolf is not, and you are not, alone. The higher power, the spiritual realm, and the positive life force: everything and all things are with us. We should acknowledge that and never forget it.

If you aren't familiar with the magical side of movement, allow an explanation of how this works. It starts with looking inside a cookie of good fortune.

What's Inside the Fortune Cookie?

Decades spent as a seeker enabled me to take account of the modern move (or better put, *collapse*) to sedentary lifestyles. Throughout this time, my mornings have been comprised of a practice of movement. The result was perfecting a fusion movement program that I continue to offer to those open to experiencing and even adopting it. Something has compelled me to develop and provide a welcome antidote to a world increasingly beleaguered by physical, mental, and emotional problems.

Peeling away the onion of health and physicality kept leading me back to the idea of freedom in movement. A search to find natural, hunter-gatherer movement directed me to the practices that originated in East Asia. This was especially true when I looked for activity that could be done on a daily basis no matter the space limitations. Much of the Asian ancient wisdom has been honed over thousands of years. So, when the working answers came from East Asia, I say I unraveled the onion with a pair of chopsticks.

Hunter-gatherers learned to hunt by watching how other animals did it. Likewise, East Asian movement is based on the flow of nature. Some arts use the movement patterns of animals. The martial arts (all of which have combat applications) use names like tiger, crane, snake, mantis, and monkey.

Bruce Lee once advised, "Empty your mind ... be formless, shapeless, like water." A dyslexic, hyperactive pre-teen, Bruce got into fights in the streets of post-World War II Hong Kong. Young Bruce began his daily meditative movement practice when his father signed him up for tai chi, which descended from qi gong. Tai chi is considered an internal martial art and is known for its health benefits including balance and relaxation. Some consider it meditative movement.

Bruce Lee—who was only an inch taller than petit Jack LaLanne—is one of the finest modern examples of the exceptional form, speed, and grace not only in the art of combat but also in the essence and expression of pure movement. Before moving to the West Coast of the United States, he was the cha-cha champion of Hong Kong.

While he's not an example of an outback hunter, he moves as gracefully as anyone who has ever been captured on film. Ballet and tap greats such as Fred Astaire, high divers such as Greg Louganis, master yogis, and Ninja martial artists are all examples of people with extraordinary skills in anatomical movement. Those old enough will remember Dr. J and Michael Jordan's feats of coordinated basketball maneuvers they deftly performed while in flight. Some will recall the on-court antics and magical ball-handling skills of the Harlem Globetrotters comedy basketball.

Bruce spent much of his time reading and writing about fitness, combat, and philosophy. He made his life not only about self-mastery but also about the purest expression of self. His workouts were varied and challenging. A slight person, he consistently sought to build power and speed. Bruce decided not to bulk up but rather to train as efficiently as possible so that he would maintain and improve his skills in martial arts. His heavy concentration on his abdomen and latissumus dorsi (lats) made his flexed body resemble a cobra. He experimented with fitness and nutrition and read widely from diverse sources. His extensive and rare library was one of his personal passions.

It's unfortunate he died at the young age of 32. Sifu Bruce certainly gave so much of himself and imparted so much in such a short time that he will long be revered. It could also be argued that he was sometimes excessive in the way he worked and trained. This resulted in broken back. From there, two pain killers per day would lead to eight, and, a few years later, early death.

"Do not pray for an easy life,
pray for the strength to endure a difficult one."
—Bruce Lee
(1940 Chinatown, San Francisco – 1973 Hong Kong)

Calisthenics

Calisthenics are bodyweight exercises such as push-ups, sit-ups, lunges, jumping jacks, squats, good-mornings, and the prostrate Superman pose. You can see them in P.E. classes, group exercise programs, military training, and athletic practices across the world. As far as we know, they have served humans for eons. We see such records in the accounts of the scribes of Ancient Greece. They are space friendly, require minimum or no props or machines, and activate the entire body.

The 20th century's popular master of calisthenics and record setter in some of them was American Jack LaLanne. Having grown up doing the movements he led from the film set of his television program, and having taken P.E. in school and college for two decades, it was easy for me to see these programs were an exceptional way to maintain fitness.

The daily program I finally embraced for myself combined what I knew of both Eastern and Western movement in what I call Bruce Lee meets Jack LaLanne. Freedom in the process allows for keeping things focused at times, allowing the mind to roam at other times. This has made for an incredible daily practice. If you add a fun-loving attitude into the mix (and some regular forays out into green areas and nature), it makes for recreation.

Daily Exercise vs. Less Frequent

The Maintenance Workout is the combo program that greets me in the morning. If you chose to try it, give it a few months and see what you think. My website features videos to purchase that demonstrate some of the exercises. It's rare that people will master new movements quickly. Patience is the most important part of all this.

If this program works for you and you wish to perfect it, then embrace it and never stop doing it. The day you sit down and think about it is the beginning of an unending mindset of blowing it off. If you avoid it once, your mind knows you can blow it off again. If you do your program each morning, there is a good chance your body will function well for the entire day.

Some of the moves I do every other day. Some of them I do every day. What I do is based on exercise science as well as innate intelligence. Done properly, you can actually feel the psychological and physiological responses that result. Since my personal lifestyle comprises lots of sitting, many of the moves are meant to increase functionality and stability.

Some people clamor after the latest news. Some of the *latest-tech* fitness crowd have recently switched to one of the *latest* of workout offerings: doing a highly intense program once per week. A company called Super Slow is marketing this *Sedentary Nation* concept across the world. A book called "Body By Science" discusses this in detail. Note that the author was an ER doc at the time he wrote the book. That means he wasn't sitting most of the day.

Dr. Doug McGuff, the ER physician, also mentions how he trains different body parts each day. He also said he adapts his workout over time. In terms of staving off atrophy and maintaining muscle mass and strength, this method does seem to produce good results.

In terms of reducing daily stress, I have found the intense and the less frequent training programs to fall short. Serotonin, a neurotransmitter that enhances mood, is released during exercise, not from sitting or standing around. Though even simple sunlight and longer days—as evidenced in the smiles during springtime in Paris—are due in part to a serotonin release. Exercise and physical activity stimulate the sympathetic nervous system.

Intermittent, intense programs seem a tad bereft in compensating for static postures, helping digestion, and tiring us out for higher quality sleep. Given certain circumstances—good biomechanics, non-sedentary lifestyle, good attitude, happy work and family life, good musculoskeletal build—such a program may work admirably. But for other people, daily exercise is far more fulfilling and life enriching. Exercise is not only about the muscle and metabolism benefits enjoyed by converts to intermittent, intense training. There is a lot of helpful biochemistry going on with daily physical movement—not the least of this involving the release of endorphins, which lower stress. Let's not forget the toxins and naturally occurring waste buildup in our bodies that is handled optimally with daily physical activity, especially rebounding. Our lymphatic system responds to this.

Dr. Joseph Mercola is the pioneer of a top wellness website with lots of helpful information. One of his online videos has him extolling the virtues of one of the speedier, less-is-more workouts. My letter to Dr. Mercola starts out, *What's the hurry in workouts? Are we in a race to get back to an 18-hour day ... indoors? When are you going to show the back-to-nature workouts? I'm available most any day ... from 5 to 7 a.m.*

An interesting study would be to test indoor exercisers for serotonin levels and compare that to outdoor exercisers. Numbers of studies have found that outdoor exercise and physical activity correlates to better mood, less workout dread, and longer workouts. The benefits of spending time outdoors—especially in nature, in fresh air, and with sunlight—are undeniable. Depression experts often attempt to stimulate an increase in serotonin levels in depression patients.

Some favor the outdoor versions of the high intensity workout. This allows for all of the benefits of being outdoors, including Vitamin D production. I have used the one-time-per-week intense protocol, going to complete exhaustion. It produced noticeable results: I put on two pounds of tissue doing it. That didn't mean I remained sedentary the other days. I still exercised; I just kept the formula of complete exhaustion down to one day per muscle group or body region per week.

Following that personal experiment, when I have energy and feel that I have recovered well, I sometimes choose to perform the complete exhaustion by muscle region every four to five days. Here's the program from last week. All workouts were outdoors, except the yoga class and some indoor warm-ups in my home.

Each day I do abs, hips, low back, structural support exercises, stretching, wrist squeezes, and some rebounding or walking. I call this daily ritual "the norm." The norm takes between 30 to 60 minutes depending on how many different exercises and reps. It typically happens at a park seeing the sunrise. Each day I take stretch breaks every bathroom break and then stretch for 2 to 5 minutes before bedtime. As needed, I perform staff acupressure (myofascial or trigger point release) for muscle pain and tension release. Sometimes I do this therapy 4 times per week. Sometimes I don't require it for several months.

1. Sunday: The norm, plus chest, arms, and shoulders. Then bodyweight squats. I felt the biceps healing until Wednesday.
2. Monday: The norm, plus neck. 5 cartwheels. 3 handstands. An evening walk around the neighborhood.
3. Tuesday: The norm at the beach at sunrise, then 3-mile run. In the evening, one hour of an official class of restorative yoga (no difficult balance positions, mostly stretching and holding of positions.)
4. Wednesday: The norm for 50 minutes in a park at sunrise. Then lunges. Then 10 minutes of back and arms with a variety of chin-ups. Then 6, 80-yard sprints up a hill. Then hit a bucket of golf balls at the range. Then jumped rope two different times during breaks from computer work.
5. Thursday: The norm at a park. Skipped rope for 5 minutes. Then bear crawling. Then 5 cartwheels.
6. Friday. 4 a.m. Long bike ride with intermittent hills. Stop at 1/3 distance to do the standing version of the norm at the beach in the moonlight. This was the first time I made this particular ride up a specific hill without getting off to walk

the bike. Finished at 7:20 a.m.

7. Saturday. Repeated Sunday plan from above.

Scientific studies may show the best formula for their particular control group. I pay attention to those findings but believe it just as important to listen to the body and get in synch with your own energy level. Since my energy level normally vacillates, especially after long periods of sitting, I tend to use the energy when it's available whether for work, exercise, or doing chores.

A sedentary job or lifestyle requires a daily counterbalance to sitting and sleeping. A walk around the neighborhood and periodic stretch breaks help, but I've found that the daily, early morning program is a necessity for me. It sets up my mind and body for a day of good possibilities. The brain gets extra oxygen during physical movement. If you want brainpower, get moving. A friend who sings suggests learning the proper techniques for singing—air support, posture, and diaphragmatic breathing—and then singing to oxygenate the brain.

Another plus of the early morning program is getting out of the house early. Human history has programmed us to be diurnal. Evolution has had humans outdoors during the day and inside at night. To be true to our nature, we should spend some time outside during the day.

I also do my outdoor program grounded to the Earth whenever possible. That means barefoot or with organic footwear like leather- or hemp-soled shoes. You can make up your own mind about being grounded to the Earth. As you contemplate this, don't just consider human longevity; use factors such as wellness and happiness. I'm a believer not only in grounding's benefit but also its necessity.

Cooking Your Groin With A Laptop

———

Previously, I mentioned I often work with a laptop on my lap. This is a negative for health but a positive for my professional and social life. In an attempt to minimize the harm, I use the following for EMFs and heat:

1. The laptop sits atop a plastic cooling plate with plenty of vent openings. I don't plug in the plate's fan, which would generate even more EMFs. These plates are available at most stores that sell laptops.

2. I place a four-inch thick, rectangular brick foam pillow under the plate and computer. I used to think that it blocked a good percentage of EMFs from heading down to my stomach and hip area. It turns out that it really only provides a padded surface with friction. If it doesn't heat you up, or if it is cooler than your laptop, that is a positive. A normal pillow smushes down and creates more heat around the groin. This more rigid brick pillow doesn't compress down, thus, the airflow can maintain room temperature. For men who want more sperm production and potency, keep that area from over heating. How to keep your "boys" cool is up to you and your boys. Some cultures have historically worn baggy outfits or loose clothing to keep things aired out as in tunics and loincloths. One health writer mentioned placing bags of ice between his thigh and his boys. "Argh, shiver me timbers."

3. Against my skin, I place a conductive grounding pad that's plugged into a grounded outlet. I plan to offer these through my website.

My computer setup isn't the perfect scenario; it's a compromise and a lousy one at that. If you have a better solution, please let me know. I do stand at a high desk but that's hard for me to do for extended periods. Movement begets movement. Sedentism begets sedentism and slouching.

The hunter-gatherers move every day. That's millions of years of daily movement, grounded to the Earth. They certainly weren't sitting in chairs for hours at a time or heading out to hunt wild game wearing rubber-soled shoes. Even when they later adopted some Westerner-style apparel, they didn't wear rubber soles until perhaps the late-20th century—see the Tarahumara sandals that were once made from leather and were later made out of a piece of tire, tied to their feet with a leather lace. A YouTube search will shed some light on these. Start with "Make huaraches (Tarahumara running sandals)." And these incredible athletes run ultramarathon distances in sandals!

What can we do to counteract sitting and standing all day?

Answer: Exercise once per day, get a desk setup that allows for different postures, both standing and sitting on a stool, and stretch every hour or at least every bathroom break.

What Would An Unrushed Tribal Counsel Say About How We Live Today?

Probably the same as the following statement from The Dalai Lama, a man who has long lived outside his country of birth due to China's heavy-handed occupation of Tibet. This quote came in an email sent right before the publishing of this book. I believe it to be a true statement.

The Dalai Lama, when asked what surprised him most about humanity, answered:

Man ... Because he sacrifices his health in order to make money. Then he sacrifices money to recuperate his health. And then he is so anxious about the future that he does not enjoy the present; the result being that he does not live in the present or the future; he lives as if he is never going to die, and then dies having never really lived. (One could add to this: often without ever realizing it.)

Absence of Stuff

Before studying the ways of the hunter-gatherers in any detail, I had already come to espouse the less-is-more doctrine of happy living. The fewer humans in the wilderness, the better off the wilderness was. The fewer cars on the road, the better the traffic circulated and the less the environment was damaged. Today there's a big push to lower our ecological footprint in whatever we do.

In my own living space, the less stuff there is to take care of, including people, the more time there is to focus on what projects I want to accomplish.* This also leaves time to spend on other normal and *essential* parts of daily living: including eating well, interacting with others and oneself, learning, resting as needed, and moving the body in a meaningful way. It may sound a bit selfish to live life as a Renaissancer (an updated and hopefully more inclusive term for

---

* There is nothing wrong with not getting married. And there is nothing wrong with not having children. People who consider that selfish might examine the reasons why they got married and had children. Most of those reasons are self-motivated, and some of it is hormonally activated. Having or not having children are both normal and natural human practices. That said, it could be argued that there is something disturbing about having children when (a) a couple doesn't have good future prospects that will allow for proper caring for themselves and their offspring, (b) the planet is severely overpopulated when you look at water supplies, fish populations, and ecosystems, and (c) reasons may be partially based on old customs (like more hands make less work), social mores, and family pressure.

Renaissance man), but perhaps not starting a family or marrying was the least selfish of my options. Since full-time philosophical and mind-body pursuits were the top priorities, I decided to focus on them.

As a writer with an active mind and imagination, also known as the very popular condition *attention deficit disorder*, I have more ideas for books and articles than I will ever be able to completely flesh out. That said, knocking out a certain number of written pages per year has long been a driving force and something that brought me the most professional fulfillment. Filling digital pages is part of my calling as a philosopher. That gets a good share of my work out of my head and into a format people can reflect on. Rewrites have allowed me to work things over with my best-informed intentions.

Here's a thought to consider. Some writers on anthropology contend humans have probably maintained a downward spiral ever since they left being hunter-gatherers. Other thinkers might suggest they were fallen people from the beginning.

Plenty of the Hunter-Gatherers Had More Downtime

A number of researchers on hunter-gatherers have found that in general—and as long as there was a good supply of food and water—bands of hunter-gatherers had more downtime, less stress, more harmony, and more fun than their neighbors and descendants who farmed. This is still evidenced today in Africa and in other parts of the world.

Tribes of quasi hunter-gatherers live nearby people of their same or similar blood lineage who have chosen to be hardworking farmers. The hunter-gatherers generally work fewer hours and are normally less prone to worry and disease than farmers. Farmers are dependent on abundant yields in order to sustain a lifestyle that includes paying for the costs of farming and, in most cases, eternal debt. You can either hunt animals that take care of themselves, or you can fence in animals and take care of them, the land, and the fence. Pathogens spread far more readily from animal to animal and from animal to human when animals are domestically raised.

Of course, these so-called "people of the land" seem to be under fire constantly by those who want their land or their strong backs—or just have mean streaks. The modern hunter-gatherer record shows that more often than not, the "people problems" faced by the hunter-gatherers have not come from within the tribe, but from the encroachment of overpopulation, greed, malfeasance, arrogance, and ignorance from outsiders.

It would not serve to dwell too long on any notions of a perpetual harmonious and peaceful existence for hunter-gatherers. One example of the harshness of Native American life can be found in Drury and Clavin's "The Heart of Everything That Is." Subtitled "The Untold Story of Red Cloud, an American Legend," this has to be one of the most compelling books I have yet to read, about one of the most captivating figures of our recent past. Drury and Clavin do admit to setting out to "spin a good yarn." But before they spun it, they did in depth research which included reading and appraising the personal journals of the residents of the forts of the U.S. Calvary. They read the accounts of both the soldiers and their wives. Knowing that written accounts don't always match the truths of the occasion, they were able to make determinations about the accuracy of the journals. Diaries are often written at times of fear and challenges. The wives of some of the soldiers did however tell accounts about the adultery that was occurring between other couples—including white soldiers and officers taking up with Native women.

Their narrative certainly captures the brutality Native American rivals sometimes inflicted upon each other. The book also details accounts of the European immigrants who were invading the Indians' territory, cheating them with false promises, feeding them rotgut whiskey, and hunting them down like animals.

At the end of my reading, a friend shared this thought: Nature is reality. To that I added: Nature can be harsh.

If nature is not reality, is a life of concrete and drywall where you choose to remain?

After reading the story of Red Cloud, it's hard to imagine any long durations of stress-free living for bands of Indians who lived in fear of having their land be taken by whites or having their village be attacked by Oglala Lakota warriors. Red Cloud and his braves were armed with modern steel knives with which they scalped and tortured their captives.

While on Red Cloud, another historical statistic took me aback. One population estimate of native peoples in North America was 19 million in 1760. It was down to 275,000 in 1920 which makes it the largest holocaust known to history. Disease, famine, war, massacre, and concentration camps (reservations) are what killed them.

Another startling piece of information came my way in a conversation about the move to intern Native Americans. The moral of the story, if you're being forced or enticed to be sedentary, watch out! This may be a way to break you down and make you subservient. Just consider the lethargy and low spirits of some of those in urban Rome in the years leading up to the fall of Rome.

Then look at the deplorable conditions on many of today's Indian reservations. The cultural collapse began by forcing Native Americans into sedentism.

Being Physically Resilient in a Global World

What can we do to thrive in an overpopulated world full of stress, disease, and disharmony?

We can get into our own heads, reset some thinking, then get out of there, into nature, and into our bodies as we reconnect with the natural fluidity of the hunter-gatherers who were hungry and had to move their bodies to get dinner. When a contact of mine read this last sentence, he reminded me they often started their day with movement … breakfast called for that.

"They didn't normally wake up to a smorgasbord of food," said a reader. "They got out of their sleeping quarters, activated their bodies, and went out and got it!"

Throwing in the Towel at Age 16

Consider for a moment the human aging process in our current era. From some innate message or through a learned convention, we somehow honor the notion that kids should be moving, playing outdoors, taking lessons in various activities, eating the right things, and napping often. Once we're adults, the subliminal thinking goes, we can work excessively or sit around all day and evening, eating and drinking whatever we fancy.

Of course we know this is not the right thing to do. But the inclination towards excessiveness witnessed in the agrarian and industrial society pervades. Dad or mom routinely work long hours or sit around a lot or both. Young people make note of this "normal" behavior and may someday mentor this unhealthful lifestyle to their kids.

Let's examine this under the lens of sedentism and ask two questions.

When does movement end? Why does it end?

It generally ends with young adulthood. And it ends mainly because we become busy with new priorities. Playtime is over.

Movement also gets replaced. Work tends to breed excessiveness in performance and work tends to be filled with sedentism. Pain and stress sets in and gets salved by a substance or an activity that relieves the stress.

The decrease in physical movement often kicks in at the same time young people begin to test their rebellious side—and begin drivers' education. Remember all of the warnings you once heard? "Don't do that, don't pick zits, don't stay up late, don't smoke, etc." At age 16, or even before, more freedom is given … or taken. Around this time, adolescents may begin a pattern of consumption of coffee, cigarettes, and alcohol. These bad habits may be considered deplorable or at least questionable for young people but may be considered perfectly acceptable for their parents. Adults are often sedentary, have busy schedules, may loathe their jobs, and suffer other pressures.

As the pressure ramps up, some of the adults and their kids find relief in drugs, both prescription and illegal. Don't forget the prescriptions sold illegally at high schools. Consuming mind-altering substances is nothing new to the planet. The lesson to remember is that you generally can't perform your daily tasks if you are perpetually high on a substance. By the same token, we can't readily and efficiently perform those tasks if we are in pain or living in depressed or manic states.

"The illegality of cannabis is outrageous, an impediment
to full utilization of a drug which helps produce
the serenity and insight, sensitivity and fellowship
so desperately needed in this increasingly
mad and dangerous world."
—Carl Sagan
(1934 Brooklyn, NY – 1996 Seattle, WA)

Here's one point of view on a very touchy and embattled subject. You of course will make your own determination. Remember that much of our recent programming has been compromised by the last 50 years of substance-aphobia. This was predominantly derived from two things: excessive drug use by citizens (including the commission of crime related to drugs) and mass hysteria generated by the government and corporate elite.

Can anyone actually sit there and suggest the intake of sufficient alcohol to cause inebriation isn't harder on the human body than processing and recovering from a buzz's worth of edible marijuana? Forget the silly 20th-century cannabis laws, let's talk the reality of pain and distress and how some of it may be mitigated. If done in a safe way and not done in a state of endless stoner-ism, marijuana may be a gift from nature that helps some get through pain, anguish, and stress. By the way, I'm an exerciser and napper, not a ganga imbiber.

$300 billion per year and pervasive ads confirms we live in a beer culture. T-shirts and TV ads are filled with beer messages. Macho men hankering for libation and escape are shown popping open aluminum tabs as they enjoy TV sports time and outback camping. The product is cheap, accessible, and provides an intoxi-cating effect. It's also a sedative—it induces sleep. Parties and evening time are filled with beer consumption.

A quick scan of the beer statistics seems to suggest a note-worthy correlation. The states that consume the most per capita are some of the most economically depressed and cold—North Dakota, New Hampshire, and Wisconsin. These three leaders are populated by consumers who drink in excess of 40 gallons of beer per year.

Is beer medicinal? It takes a lot of energy to digest alcohol; therefore, for most of us, it is likely not good medicine. Naturally grown marijuana is far easier on human biology. If a friend was dying of cancer or was clinically depressed, could you accept their use of cannabis? Even their partial stoner-ism? If this is you, consider opting for the edible organic marijuana over the typically prescribed unnatural, synthesized pharmaceuticals. If you do imbibe in herb, avoid lighting up. It's better for us to avoid inhaling hot, unfiltered smoke of any kind.

So, if you want throat and lung health, avoid the doobies. If you are in pain, dying of cancer, some doctors may prescribe morphine. Do you know what morphine does to your body? It backs you up. It stops peristalsis. Do you want to be constipated while you are numbed out and dying?

The human body is one of the most incredible instruments ever designed. It responds beautifully to sound sleep as well as to natural movement patterns like dancing; running in thin-soled, earthed footwear; bear crawling on our hands and feet (not on our knees like toddlers—a bit hard on the joints and bones); and bearing our own weight on horizontal bars or supporting ourselves during low-impact exercises like push-ups on suspension belts.

Biomechanically efficient exercises have been some of the most effective in creating athletic superstars, in preventing injury, and in rehabilitating people from injury. Basketball's retired and once largest and most dominant center is Shaquille O'Neal, who hails from my home state of New Jersey. The 320- to 340-pound center credits his core exercise strength training with healing some of his nagging injuries and prolonging his phenomenal career, which left him as the sixth highest scorer in NBA history.

Now that he's in retirement from his high-intensity pro career, one would hope that Shaq would avoid the trappings of a predomi-nantly desk and car lifestyle. Nearly every body-worker and physical therapist shares this with their patients. "We weren't meant to spend long periods of time sitting and standing in static positions." They know, because they don't thrive while sitting. As they stand and engage their bodies, therapists tend to get energized during the work day. The body generally responds well to being used.

How hard is it to change your posture, especially if it's a perpetually sitting position? How hard is it to change whatever repetitive or detrimental posture you may have? Try doing some postural improvement for at least a portion of the day. Treat your-self not like a boxed lunch or machine, but like a work of art. If we work on our physical balance, we gain both physical and emotional balance. The statistics show that aged and fragile seniors who fall and break some things tend to die within six months. Shouldn't we help seniors with exercise classes, assistance, remodeling the living space, and learning about falling?

Treating ourselves with care helps provide the positive posture, and the fortitude of mind to treat other residents of the world, all living things, and even the path we stand on, with respect and gratitude.

Treat yourself with respect. And then play that out to others and the planet.

Easy Takeaways

1. Get fit and functionally strong. Then emulate some of the movement patterns of the hunter-gatherers. When you're fit and able, pretend you're Tarzan running to save animals and Jane. Go around objects—trees, posts, road signs, cones, and other objects. Flow with your surroundings. This is not only fun, it's natural to mix up the direction of your running.

2. Rest when needed, or celebrate and commune when the food acquisition and chores have been accomplished. Celebrate while working for the food.

3. "It's better to wear away than to rust away." Some movement, even if it's repetitive, might be considered better than no movement.

4. Unravel the modern onion with a pair of chopsticks. Dine more slowly and eat less. Look into the movement practices of East Asians.

5. If a program works for you and you wish to perfect it, embrace it and never stop doing physical movement—not even for a day.

6. Our body is one of the most incredible instruments ever designed. Treat it like a work of art.

Chapter 7

Downtime

Downtime (original meaning): the time when a machine of production broke down.

That definition has grown to encompass systems and manufactured technologies that break down, which means production halts.

Age of Sedentism version of the word: the time a human can spend quietly away from the grind. This could include surfing the Net and watching a flat screen movie.

Natural-Path version: time spent away from systems of technology, production, and busyness in general. This could include reading an actual book, going for a walk, daydreaming, and resting.

The Fight for the Almighty Last Say

Who's fighting for control in the business of health and wellness?

Many leading scholars and those educated in medicine have seen incomes grow at unprecedented rates over the past 60 years.

Some of these professions are now seeing their career territory in flux and possible jeopardy. Downsizing and budget cuts have impacted the entire economy.

Information is readily available on the Net, and surfers can peruse the long and short of millions of topics. As relates to providers of information on health, there's a noticeable and relatively contentious turf war for paying consumers, blog followers, and book-buying believers. Then there are the research studies. Publications are so hungry to publish new studies that it becomes a virtual feeding frenzy. Some of the studies are offered openly on the Internet and some carry a subscription or access fee.

The infotainment sources seem the hungriest for new health news. About this, one health speaker related, "The media never met a new study it didn't like." New studies create news and initiate interest. If the study contradicts an older accepted finding, even more attention is generated.

For the most part, consumers have access to the same studies as physicians. Compared to the general public, physicians no doubt have superior schooling and background in reading studies. But across the planet there is a growing interest in all parts of knowledge and cultural trends. People are reading and talking more on health matters and are becoming more aware. If you ask normal people about their cholesterol, they might give you very detailed answers. They may also know their body fat percentage, the side effects of medicines they have never taken, the current increasing trend in autoimmune diseases, and the latest news on omega-3 fatty acids. As I write this paragraph, I just received an email regarding the Weston Price Foundation's March Against Monsanto. I doff my hat to all of that.

If you have had the occasion to read through one, you may agree that the published health research studies are often long and technical. To someone who wants *the skinny*, rather than reading the studies themselves, it's generally far less complicated to read the journalistic articles about the research's findings. For me, it's best when I can read a summary of several decades or even centuries of thought on a specific subject. When done with that, I then consider what might be the sensible, natural approach to the topic. The Internet and books have been immensely helpful in providing entertaining and helpful summaries of health information.

In the early 1990s, I had the good fortune to spend time with a physician in her final years of oncology residency. This offered a firsthand view of how inundated she was with photocopies of cancer treatment studies. The piles of studies were so thick that it was difficult to access the useful information. Then came improvements in the Internet, PDFs, and easier key-word searching.

Busy physicians and scientists often have hectic schedules, potentially with cell phones ringing after hours and grant proposal and research study deadlines always approaching. Now for the ultimate health question: "How balanced are the lives these highly educated people are leading?"

A first thing to consider: Are they sedentary during the workday? Most practicing physicians are not. They tend to be on their feet and moving most of the day. So at least they're not desk potatoes. Depending on their tasks, lab scientists and researchers may or may not be sedentary in the workplace. Lab work these days is often seated, often using a computer—head tilted, back hunched, hips smushed, and nerves not firing well.

More workplace things to consider: Is there easy and affordable access to good food?

Who has more favorable access to healthful food, the doctor, the worker in the big commercial complex, or Joe the plumber who stops for lunch in a town that has healthful options? Whose job provides more movement? Whose job might allow for a post-lunch nap in a van parked under a tree?

Remember that busyness, deadlines, and meetings can easily cause stress. When we consider the lives of "health experts," remember that many suffer reduced periods of time in which to take care of themselves. If that is indeed the case, consumers with time on their hands for wellness have the chance to live equally healthful or more healthful lives than the so-called experts simply by embracing the balanced, natural approach.

Never forget that sound sleep is as important as physical activity. Of course we all make compromises in certain areas, and we are unable to do everything as well as we'd like. Even if wellness is a priority, would you sacrifice it to accomplish a specific goal? Jesus, Joan of Arc, Gandhi, Indira Gandhi, Martin Luther King, and perhaps even Steve Jobs all opted for a path that made a tremendous impact. This path, in each of these cases, ended with the ultimate sacrifice.

"Oh, yes. I'd do it all again; the spirit is willing yet;
I feel the same desire to do the work but the flesh is weak.
It's too bad that our bodies wear out while our
interests are just as strong as ever."

—An aged Susan B. Anthony, Civil Rights,
Temperance Movement, and Woman's Suffrage
(1820 Adams, Mass. – 1906 Rochester, N.Y.)

Sleep and Morning Dread

Does it make any sense that so many people wake up in prolonged grogginess in the morning?

What is a good night's sleep supposed to do? It's supposed to be rejuvenating, not cause a morning of low energy. I've been guilty of morning dread myself, not always waking up raring to go. In fact, there were plenty of times in my youth when I used to sleep in past normal breakfast hours when I could. Adolescence is often a challenging experience, with daily commitments, stresses, and the body's growth spurts. Young people are known to be less tired than adults in the early part of the night. This has to do with their circadian rhythms and a later at night increase in melatonin levels. This means there is a tendency to stay up past the recommended hour that would correspond to their morning schedules. Knowing this, some have lobbied schools to begin classes later in the morning.

Obviously, bedtime hour is the main determinant for wakeup hour. After figuring out how sleep works within a balanced and productive life, I now generally go to sleep early and wake up ready for my morning routine. The aging process, together with age-altered melatonin levels, certainly has a lot to do with this. The freedom, exhilaration, and earthing provided by my early morning routine makes it one of the best parts of the day. (Again, "earthing" means bare feet or leather soles on the ground to conduct and synchronize with the electric charge of the Earth.)

Efficiency is also important in managing sleep time. When things are clicking, when anxiety isn't causing your heart to race, how soon do you fall asleep? For siestas and nighttime sleep, I normally go from eyes closed to fully asleep in a short, few minute's time. I don't think it makes sense to have a researcher hook up the sensation wires to my cranium and heart to test this. It might mess me up. Sleep is too valuable a personal love to disrupt.

The Ever-Evolving Great Foot Debate

Before some of us think of going to sleep, we spend some time on our feet, walking or running. These are two physical activities that have seen some changes in the West's new millennium. Numbers of people have removed their shoes and have taken on barefoot physical activity. Some with success, some with bone bruises and glass shards.

A number of podiatrists and sports medicine doctors have spoken out against the barefoot running movement. This movement also includes the thin-soled or limited-sole athletic shoe. This story was popularized by Christopher McDougal's best-selling book, "Born to Run." This captivating book demonstrates how wellness sometimes worked before the advent of modernism.

Its rich back-story features some remarkable American runners who travel to Mexico to race the Tarahumara, perhaps the best varying elevation trail runners in the world. With all the elements of engaging storytelling this book cohesively documents part of the history of modern running. It also describes what seems the most natural approach to running whose roots, if you can historically imagine, predate Nike, Asics, Adidas, and modern orthotics.

In a videotaped interview, the journalist and author argues for the barefoot cause. In what looks to McDougal like a move to protect their turf, a number of podiatrists and sports medicine doctors started making claims against the barefoot movement. This, McDougal asserts, came with no accepted or authenticated medical studies backing their claims. In one section of his book, the author mentions the scarcity of medical problems enjoyed by the Tarahumara who live in Mexico's Copper Canyon. These groups of Mexican Indians have been *"hiding out"* since the age of Spain's Conquistadors and have long practiced what we term *extreme distance running.* Even their seasoned citizens are known to run great distances … like 70 miles at age 70. *Impresionante, no es verdad?*

Many members of this tribal group live in remote areas and live simply, like their ancestors did. This puts them in a direct connection with nature. Those who live far from the sedentary villages are said to have no diabetes, heart conditions, depression, colon cancer, or foot-related repetitive injuries. Their biggest threat comes from the closest sedentary towns where resident Tarahumara face apathy and processed foods. Other threats to the outback Tarahumara come from the Mexican drug cartels who have sought out the most inaccessible areas to grow and traffic drugs.

A stirring element of the story is how the Tarahumara are said to run with joy, not with the grimacing faces of exhaustion and disquiet sometimes seen on untold numbers of the hyper-programmed busy creatures we see on our roads, tracks, and marathon events.

The outback Tarahumara, McDougal affirms, rarely need doctors and don't know what a podiatrist is. They run in thin sandals, land on the forefoot, and glide through the air like gazelles. Their smooth strides are more reminiscent of Olympic sprinter Jessie Owens in 1936 than the American joggers of our recent past who were often trained to land heel first. Heel-first landing, proponents of the forefoot landing propose, is contrary to how proper running should be done. "All you have to do," says McDougal, "is watch a five-year-old run. They know how to run, and run with joy."

The more people learn how to move themselves properly, with posture and efficiency, hopefully the fewer appointments for orthotics, plantar fasciitis, and shin splints they will require.

Foot Problems

Some shoe or running stores offer to spend a fair amount of time with their customers to fit them for molded inserts. Dr. Julia Overstreet, advises other doctors on her YouTube video called "Plantar Fasciitis explained by a Podiatrist." She states that plantar fasciitis is a mechanical problem that requires a mechanical solution. Dr. Overstreet suggests two different over-the-counter sole inserts to try. Both companies she mentions have orthotics available for under $50 a pair.

There are often good solutions found using Western medicine. Who would argue that it would be better to see the medical system utilized more for prevention than repair?

If it continues to gain converts, the barefoot movement will directly impact the running-shoe industry and the healthcare industry. This is not to say it's for everyone. For someone whose gait is amiss, barefoot endurance running (or any repetitive, high impact endeavor whether barefoot or shod) is not recommended. Walking and running properly may come naturally for some, but for others it's somewhere between a tall order and an impossibility.

During my time as a part-time professional mascot, my podiatrist was helpful in showing me how to walk properly and providing me with sport-orthotics. Another practitioner who works in biomechanics had me place a piece of soft foam between my big toe and second toe to promote pressing off those two metatarsals. Some of this helped to permanently change the way I walk. But, despite our better proactive efforts, it's not always easy to change instinctive or long-adopted biomechanics. I certainly walk better than before, but my gait is far from perfect.

Someone has to teach proper walking to those who lack natural good steps or biomechanical know-how. I see kids walking with their parents on the beach. Many of the little tikes have substantial problems with their arches and striding gait. That should be the time those issues are addressed—when we're young. Improving your gait should prove fruitful to your path of wellness. When you stabilize your foot and kinetic chain posture, walking will become a joy. If it's a joy, I'd call it a form of natural-path downtime.

Thanks for the Memories

Many of the companies that finance significant portions of the research that goes into the science and delivery of healthcare stand to lose revenues if people live more like they did before the advent of modernism. If we looked at how many times the vast majority of our great-grandparents called in sick or just decided to sleep in, we might be able to determine who was healthier and more motivated. When they were unable do their jobs in the old days, it's likely they were really down for the count. This isn't to suggest one heads in to work and operates at 10 percent capacity and focus, but that the olden days had lots of resilient citizens.

The average American lifespan in 1909 was 47. At first glance, that sounds like those folks had much tougher, shorter lives. It's not that simple. The figure is misleading because it counts people who died while children. Child mortality decreased significantly over the course of the 20th century—welcome news. Most adults, however, weren't dropping off at age 47. They lived longer lives, and some would argue, "much more fulfilling lives than we live today." Don't forget, we are the medicated nation (aka Prozac nation). Our generation is known to take psychotropic drugs and visit counselors and life coaches because we experience disturbances and challenges we cannot seem to handle very well on our own. And many of us don't have the support of a caring, extended family living close by. Numbers of those who do currently live in proximity to their family confess to wanting to get as far away as possible.

With the rise of the "sandwich generation," more and more, people are caring for their children as well as their parents. Grandparents have nieces and nephews and even ex-spouses of their kin living with them. As homes combine, those in need of care are helped by family and friends who may live under the same roof and also act as caregivers. There is certainly nothing wrong with this trend. In known history, this is the way it has always been. Families and friends, and tribal people, have always collaborated and assisted. In 1910, this was common as well as essential to their survival.

Longevity is a statistic we frequently read about. Forgetting about longevity, which group shows the need for more medical care in terms of ordinary living ... people in 1910 or people today? Not counting childbirth, epidemics, accidents, poisonings, non-potable water, and poorly preserved food, who needed more appointments because they were simply unwell due to things like poor diets, overmedication, and sedentism?

A recent statistic said the average American had 12 prescriptions filled per year. Does that sound good to you? In my estimation, the prior generations were the healthier group. One of the primary reasons for this is because many lived in the rural areas. As previously stated, remember that many regions had rural directly adjacent to the big cities at the turn of the 20th century. Rural wasn't too far from Manhattan back in 1910. In fact, New York City's surrounding areas were filled with farms.

Rural meant fresh air, time outdoors, fresh produce, less EMFs, less sound and light pollution, lots of physical labor, and sounder sleep. It also meant working and eating meals as families. Spending quality time with family is incredibly beneficial. John Robbins, in his book "Healthy at 100," lists family time, including grandparents' involvement with grandkids, as one of the principal drivers for excellent health and longevity. These are cultural practices embraced by the centenarians of Okinawa and Sardinia.

As I plodded my way through the fact-filled books on wellness like those by John Robbins and Dan Buettner, and books by physicians, researchers, and psychologists, I found themes that mostly corroborated what had long been my lifestyle philosophy. But occasionally I found points of view that caused me to stop dead in my tracks. The following is an example.

A Food Shocker

Maui's Wailuku Library is one on the list of many libraries around the globe that have provided me very exceptional periods of peaceful writing and inquiry. They're perfect places for downtime and reconnecting with self. As a matter of fact, besides a chance to sit around at one of the Babe Ruth, Lou Gehrig World Series' games, a quiet library would have to be one of my first choices of sitting spaces. This specific locale near the municipal buildings of Maui is a dandy. Built in 1928, the Wailuku Library is listed on the National

Register of Historic Places. I closed my laptop as I took a break from my writing one winter's day on the volcanic-born landmass. Then came something that has become a personal custom. Another library patron had left a magazine on the table. It was so fascinating a publication, I couldn't put it down. Among other interesting pieces, the Utne Reader held an article entitled "In Praise of Fast Food: We need a culinary ethos that comes to terms with industrialized food."

How remarkable, I thought. *Come to terms, hum?* Well now, what would this particular writer say to the unconverted, true-food proponents whose longstanding culinary ethos would seek to throw most of this denatured and nutrient-deficient "industrial crap" into the hazardous materials dumpsite? Would she at least vote for disbanding the kissing cousins in the food oversight boards? The FDA and Big Ag.

This particular article attempted to and succeeded in casting doubt in the notion old-school eating was somehow more natural. Here is part of "The Gastronomica Reader" by Rachel Laudan that was excerpted in the Utne article. It is listed here for critique purposes.

For our ancestors, natural was something quite nasty. Natural often tasted bad. Fresh meat was rank and tough, fresh fruits inedibly sour, fresh vegetables bitter. Natural was unreliable. Fresh milk soured; eggs went rotten. Everywhere seasons of plenty were followed by seasons of hunger. Natural was also usually indigestible. Grains, which supplied 50 to 90 percent of the calories in most societies, have to be threshed, ground, and cooked to make them edible. So to make food tasty, safe, digestible, and healthy, our forebears bred, ground, soaked, leached, curdled, fermented, and cooked naturally occurring plants and animals until they were literally beaten into submission. They created sweet oranges and juicy apples and non-bitter legumes, happily abandoning their more natural but less tasty ancestors. They built granaries, dried their meat and their fruit, salted and smoked their fish, curdled and fermented their dairy products, and cheerfully used additives and preservatives—sugar, salt, oil, vinegar, lye—to make edible foodstuff.[32]

I encourage everyone to read the complete article whose link is found in my endnotes and to consider the work of those like Luther Burbank whose innovative natural techniques improved the taste and nutritive value of vegetables and fruits. Laudon is quite observant: Who could refute that preserving food is imperative, especially in a world of populated areas, seasonal changes, distance shipping, and local food scarcity? The degree of preservation and use of chemicals and radiation are what concerns many health proponents. Who wants a piece of fruit that was sprayed with chemicals, picked too early, and shipped too far, only to be stored for too long?

Of course many of the places we inhabit don't possess the soil, weather, or available nearby land. Fresh food is often especially hard to come by. (Ever been to Vegas? Despite the irrigation, it's still a rocky desert.) But there's a big difference between *legitimately* preserving food and today's practice of loading food with sodium, sugar, and fat because of their taste properties which are incredibly addictive.

Why couldn't we be happy with the tastes of our grandparents' era? Tabletop seasonings such as salt and pepper and A1 Steak Sauce worked fine. Why did we have to change all that and cram all the taste inside the food? Are we too feeble to lift a small bottle of seasoning? Or are we simply programmed to clamor for injected food?

By and large, modern factory-farmed food and agribusiness-farmed produce is devoid of integrity. The way we provide food today is generally not healthful for nature, animals, or us. To recall the vocalizing style of the anti-broccoli man himself, George H. W. Bush (the dad who was a WWII veteran), old-school eating and living ... good; agribusiness run amok ... bad!

Here's a well-scripted reply to an email I sent out to a group of my wellness contacts with a link to the Laudan article. Isaac Osborne, a posture alignment therapist and avid reader on health issues, sent me a stinging response. "Are we supposed to thank food science and industry for our longevity? Okay, thank you. Are we supposed to thank food growers and producers for contributing toward genetically modified, pesticide ridden, unnatural plastic food junk? Isn't it possible to have modern conveniences while preserving the integrity of plants and animals?

"Of course, but we'd have to change the paradigm to do that. We are paying a high price with disease and dysfunction in our bodies for that convenience. There are many symptoms in society that are on the rise. Childhood obesity, teenage arthritis, Alzheimer's, ADD and ADHD, diabetes, and many more that were not as prevalent 20 to 30 years ago. They are getting worse, in part because the food is getting worse.

"The lives of indigenous cultures do revolve around foraging, fishing, and farming. But food was the *whole* tribe's responsibility. Also, there are many groups who were so efficient that they had time for numbers of other activities. Take the Hawaiians for example. Their farming and fishing techniques were so efficient that they had time for surfing, art, big luaus, and downtime. A good read, if you want more information, is an old book from 1939 called 'Nutrition and Physical

Degeneration' by Weston Price."[33] The title itself pushes some buttons.

Even a grand thinker such as dentist and health theorist Weston Price is not without his detractors. But rather than get into a long discussion about that, I'd like to again remind that the latest information available should not cause you to stop considering practical questions on your own—and tapping into your intuition. The latest information shouldn't automatically become sound-minded truths to implement in your lifestyle.

The Utne subtitle itself is spine tingling: "We need a culinary ethos that comes to terms with industrialized food." Yes, "comes to terms with." Okay, we humanoids foraged for millions of years, farmed for about 12,000, and now have factory farmed and factory produced for a handful of generations. Now we're overpopulated, polluting, bored, and causing climate change. So, what are the terms? Do we stay the course and wind up, as one author puts it, extinct because of human excess? In her book, "The Sixth Extinction, An Unnatural History," Elizabeth Kolbert points to humans as the cause of the next great extinction. Do we need an acceptable ethos for that or should we be responsible stewards of the planet and our own shortsighted excesses?

"The Latest" Trumps Good Sense

Here's a case in point of a strange way we are teaching our students—in this case, a doctoral student. One suggestion I received from a PhD student who viewed some of my fitness philosophy was to "quote studies released within two to three years prior to my publication. That way," he said, "people in *my* field will take the knowledge seriously."

His statement makes all the sense in the world when you

consider who is funding universities: people, countries, and companies that want to create new waves of things to sell, including downloadable PDFs of research studies.* His statement also holds no water when you talk to experts on ancient philosophies. Are we smarter and happier today than people were in the past? Certainly not all of the past.

It's absurd that students educated in the new millennium are taught that new knowledge is so much more important than older knowledge, furthering the awkward notion that the latest-greatest is generally better than timeworn wisdom.

> *"To know by rote is not to know; it is to retain*
> *what one has entrusted to his memory. That which*
> *a man rightly knows he is the true disposer of,*
> *without looking at the model or glancing at his book."*
> —Michel de Montaigne
> (1533 – 1592, born and died in Bordeaux region of France)

By the way, Montaigne was a Renaissance author revered among his peers and writers to this day. In his speech and writing he had an incredible ability to mix knowledge with personal anecdotes. In my graduate studies program in French we learned that Montaigne had a German *précepteur*, his personal instructor of all things. The

---

* During a radio interview of Abbas Milani, Director of Iranian Studies, Stanford, Dr. Milani revealed that Iran, under the Shah in the 1970s, gave millions of dollars to MIT to educate and train nuclear engineers and physicists for Iran's nuclear program. The Commonwealth Club radio program. February 2011. This is but one example of a university receiving funding from questionable benefactors. Are some of our temporary or potential allies questionable benefactors? Most certainly!

educator was a doctor who spoke no French. Horstanus spoke only Latin to the boy and would wake the young Michel by wafting a feather above his head or touching it against his skin. Is that a more pleasurable awakening than the cock crowing in the yard or the garbage collector in the alley?

Living Off the Grid

There is a current move to live more "naturally."

Old friends of mine who work big-city jobs in rainy London Town still love watching reruns of American TV's classic "The Waltons." It's a program that appeals to their sentimental look back to the old days. The Walton family faced many challenges during the Great Depression, but they always seemed to work together, help each other in the community, and pull through. Have you heard of living off the grid? Or urban homesteading?*

Living off the grid means not needing, or needing very little in the way of, public power sources and public water.

Urban homesteading has given larger residential lots a facelift … and some new sounds. From the back alley, a passerby may note that noise and pollution of lawnmowers and leaf blowers has been replaced by the soft neighs of a few goats. Yes, goats. The urban homesteaders plant sustainable gardens and raise smaller critters like chickens, game hens, guinea fowl, fish, bees, goats, and pigs. None of this is easy, but it is certainly a more "earthy" way to go than landing distance-shipped food at the airport's tarmac and shopping at the conglomerate's mega food store. If you're retired, the garden time might just become a principal driving force in

---

* Aka hobby farming or small-scale farming.

your life.

We all need something to do. Men are known to move into retirement and die in the first year. Without the bonding that women seem better equipped for, many Western men tend to stay more on their own during retirement. This can lead to channel flipping, overeating, sedentism, stress, and boredom. Would you want to spend your retirement in the hereafter?

I have been following the urban homesteading movement for some time. No video clip has been more compelling than the one sent to me about the Jules Dervaes family backyard farm—it's in Los Angeles. The retired Jules says, "Growing your own food is a dangerous act because you're in danger of becoming free."

Jules feeds his 4-person family and the remaining produce is sold. His adult kids share in the farm work. Their work on the residential lot makes $20,000 per year on 4,000 square feet of garden. That equates to 6,000 pounds of food on a tenth of an acre urban farm which houses two goats, four chickens, and a number of ducks.[34]

A number of soon-to-be retirees of the corporate world have confided to me they can't wait to get away from modernism. They can't wait to move to a rural or remote area and live *off the grid* with their own solar water pumps, eco-friendly buildings like yurts, and organic gardens.

Are scores of work-a-day 40 to 60-ish folks ready to swap golf clubs and barbells for pitchforks and sickles? Are they ready to close down their cable TV accounts, buy some non-GMO seeds, and join the ranks of the urban homesteader?

So many of us are frustrated with how the big machine works. Some news even boggles the mind. I take periodic runs in Santa Barbara past lemon orchards that produce high quality fruit. I met a former administrator in a local agricultural cooperative who informed me, "Most of those lemons get shipped to Japan."

"And our lemons come from … ?" I asked.

With a disappointed grin he said, "Wholesalers store it outside our county, let it sit until a grocer orders it, and then ship it to us."

"Meaning we sink our teeth into fruit that's not that fresh?" I pressed.

"Could be fresh, may not be so fresh."

"Is that capitalism or unsustainable lunacy?" I asked.

"I've been asking that question for decades," he admitted.

A few months after that, I visited a friend in Hawaii. Since the airport was nearby the mega centers, we stopped by a big store on the first day to pick up some fruits and vegetables. While we were in line, we noticed mold on some of the apples, right in the hole that leads to the core.

"They're last year's apples," my friend told me.

"Are you sure?" I asked him. "You mean last season, right? Today is Christmas Eve."

This friend lived and worked on an organic farm for several years and knows a good deal about produce. "What I mean is, they're old apples. Grocers often buy things at a discount. The [chain's employee] buyer … well, it's that person's job not only to find the best produce but the produce they can get a deal on."

We hear of buying local and hiring local. Who wouldn't be for that? But hardly anyone likes to pay double at the farm or market what it costs in the store … and buying organic, and even just buying healthful produce and goods, is certainly not cheap. Our smarter ancestors would buy local when they could. They wanted their neighbor's profits to cycle back through the community. So no, I'm not opposed to finding my answers back in time especially when they're more sensible.

The intention is to provide a view into the past and also give mindset and lifestyle tips so we in the busy, modern era can be fulfilled, happy, and well as we do our best to thrive in today's culture.

Anthropology 101 and Movement

Mentioning archeology and anthropology is likely to open up a can of worms no matter how you frame the discussion. Once, when I mentioned the words "hunter-gatherers" to a learned man who works in medicine, he rolled his eyes. Mentioning movement also creates a stir. Once, when I mentioned my philosophy to a retired physician who parties a bit and admits to taking medicine to alleviate the woes, he countered, "People don't have to do much movement." In his mind he was currently doing okay without it.

Rather than instigate angst, such discussions of historical references should be entertained with openness. Reading on subjects such as anthropology and archeology for several decades, I am always impressed by innovative thinking that uses the historical evidence, combines it with all of the schools of learning—including psychology and sociology—and comes up with sensible hypotheses. The conclusions are quite another story. It's hard to get unwavering accuracy and closure on anything, especially when it relates to really old bones and not-so-old "ancient" texts. Ancient religious texts, starting with the Pyramid texts of Ancient Egypt, are only about 4,300 years old.

Scientists postulate that early human types began by gathering food and scavenging carcasses that other predatory animals had killed. Eventually, early humanoids added hunting to their scavenging and gathering in what became known as the subsistence method.

Then, about two million years ago, a big climatic change occurred, and the forests in Africa turned to grasslands—savannas. When game animals moved on, tribes followed.

Much later, around 28,000 B.C., the physically stronger and heavier Neanderthal species (whose bones have thus far only been found in Eurasia) disappeared. But not without leaving a trace … in us. Research has recently determined that today, non-African modern humans have somewhere between 1 and 4 percent Neanderthal DNA. The interbreeding hypothesis of Neanderthals and Homo sapiens was finally proven in the new millennium.

To this day, we still don't know why the Neanderthals disappeared. One theory posits that, compared to Homo sapiens, the Neanderthals may have had more limited speech ability due to the position of their hyoid bone and the shorter length of their larynx.

Oral communication has been one of the main methods of teaching and organizing the societies of Homo sapiens. If one species had better ways to transmit information and innovative methodologies, they would have a definite survival advantage. The brains of Neanderthals, according to their cranial capacity, were slightly larger than the Homo sapiens, so according to the limited speech theory, they were potentially less limited in thinking than in speech.

Don't judge too soon, though. DNA evidence seems to contradict the limited speech theory. According to a team of researchers led by Johannes Krause of the Max Planck Institute for Evolutionary Anthropology in Leipzig, Germany, Neanderthals shared the same *FOXP2* gene—the speech-enabling gene—as our Homo ancestors.

Another extinction theory starts with the challenges

Neanderthals may have had in obtaining food. Some posit their thicker bodies required huge numbers of calories per day. As far as calorie count, 5,000 is an amount a number of scientists seem to agree on, while still others suggest only 100 to 250 more calories than Homo sapiens, which could put the number in the two thousands.

Daniel Lieberman, in his book on human evolution, discusses the premise that Neanderthals likely had less complex wiring and frontal lobe development than Homo sapiens. This may have made our Homo ancestors better cooperators and better inventors. Might we have been "culturally" and communally superior to other ancient humans? The artwork our progenitors left may suggest just that. Prehistoric campsites, Lieberman attests, show that Neanderthals, "lacked modern humans' tendencies to invent new tools, adopt new behaviors, and express themselves as much using art."[35]

Neanderthals were squatter and had larger torsos and limbs than Homo sapiens. Though their hands were basically the same size.

Man vs. Ape

This leads to another question: Who would have won in a fight to the death?

Individually, in one-on-one unarmed combat, it's likely a Neanderthal would have kicked a Homo sapiens' butt. First, their craniums with the extended brow ridge are better adapted to take a blow to the face. Coming from years spent in martial arts and grappling, I, a tall sapling of grappling, will admit to having been at times tossed around with ease by those who had thicker, more powerful bodies, especially those who were squatter, more Neanderthalesque. Though, I have also out-fought and submitted plenty of physically imposing opponents.

Mass, strength, and balance do tend to help the larger or wider grapplers. With equal balance and stability, the larger mass imparts tremendous force on a smaller mass. Given relatively similar skill levels and cunning, if the wider body can dominate the smaller person before running out of energy, the wider body wins.

If the fight drags on, the one with less muscle mass may see their chances increase. Endurance is a significant part of combat capacity. We know that it takes a lot of energy to pump blood through a body, especially during a physically demanding session at high intensity. This is one of the reasons why many competitors in combat arts (such as mixed martial arts fighters) condition themselves to be at their optimal weight. Depending on the weight class and their payday arrangements, fighters do have an optimal fight weight. To remain at this optimal weight, many fighters may avoid bulking up with added fat and muscle tissue. A fighter or endurance athlete wants to use their fuel to create energy for their sport, not to pump blood through all of that hungry living tissue. It's unlikely today's bulked-up football players could play both offense and defense in a sustained play-ground-style game with no TV timeouts—even if they were mainlining Red Bull. They'd simply run out of juice.

Even though today's smaller combat fighters sometimes outlast or outmaneuver larger fighters, it's probably unlikely that unarmed, individual Homo sapiens were consistently able to do that to Neanderthals.

The following is an outlandish example to illustrate the simple point of superior force, but consider it anyway. How would Bruce Lee or Mike Tyson have fared, even armed with a knife or a club, against a well-fed alpha-male gorilla or even a sleepy female gorilla?

Not very well. Or even against a chimpanzee or bonobo? Any top MMA fighter would have his arm dislocated and neck snapped in short order by even the smaller of Great Apes.

It might be accurate to draw the power line at small apes like gibbons. If you compare these ultra-tiny simians to bigger, stronger humans, it's probably a different story. Entering the UFC Octagon (cage fighting) in a Pay Per View fight, a tiny, little fellah like the gibbon might choose best to run (or climb) for his life ... or use quick-biting teeth.

Primatologist Frans de Waal writes about man versus ape. Some consider chimps small since on all fours they only come up to our knees, he reminds us. "But they can almost fly up even a branchless tree. No human being can do that."

Scientists have measured the arm-pulling strength of a male chimpanzee at five times that of an athletic young man. "And since apes fight with four hands, they are impossible to beat ... even if they are prevented from biting."[36]

Since de Waal's 2005 book, however, other tests have been done which place bonobo strength at double in jumping tests. Perhaps not five times more blast off, but when it comes to jumping, double at least. Some of the science suggests it's our physical control that subjects us to weaker strength; whereas chimps have more of an all or nothing use of their powerful force.[37]

A look at basic evolution may provide the final wrap up. Evolution made us stronger of mind and made simians stronger of body. We survived with brains that put us atop the food chain while simians have to hide in the trees. Though humans have to hide in trees at times. A native of northern Italy told me he hide in the trees with his brothers. This was in the late 1940s, at night coming home from work in the village. Prowling wolves sent the boys to the branches. Even as young men, the boys knew they had far greater climbing ability than the lupi—which is the plural wolves in Italian. After analyzing what we know, some have concluded that as a coordinated group, Homo sapiens might have out-communicated and out-thought the Neanderthals.

The Neanderthal body type—squatter with wider pelvises—suggests they weren't as adept at running and walking long distances as the Homo sapiens. Thus, the heavily muscled Neanderthals were less able to employ *persistence hunting*—running animals until they keel over. Their large size also restricted their success in other methods that required distance traveling and sustained fast walking and running.

Did our slightly taller, thinner bodies enable us to better react to climate changes? Paul Mellars of Cambridge University wrote an article stating so. "The evidence is here that modern humans could cope with cold conditions better than the Neanderthals thanks to culture and technology—for instance, with better clothing, better fire control, and perhaps better shelters."[38]

This ability to weather the weather by no means suggests that Homo sapiens have an easy road to perpetuity. The Neanderthals successfully survived, often through ice ages, for some 100,000 years. Other estimates put their existence at far greater time spans: even 350,000 years.

When the Homo sapiens appeared on the hunt (or the gather) perhaps 200,000 years ago, they began by grunting in Africa and eventually wound up singing for audiences at Carnegie Hall. Along the way, with their own two feet, they had to hunt wild game—often much speedier prey. One hypothesis is that our predecessors thrived in part due to their (and our) ability at distance running.

These hunting hominids were able to cause quadrupeds, like antelopes and zebras, to gallop at length, resulting in their keeling over with heat exhaustion.[39] And if push came not just to shove but to well thought-out battle, it's possible a group of us could have defeated the Neanderthals due to our genetic and evolutionary gifts. It's possible we were able to outrun, outtalk, and probably outfight the stronger but less mobile Neanderthals. It's likely the fights were not won with superior brute force but perhaps with technique, technology, and organization.

When it came to eating, we didn't have any problem carving up keeled-over wild game to feed the family. Those Homo sapiens who had access to fruits, vegetables, grains, nuts, roots, and grubs likewise made a feast of those.

Antelopes Can't Pant and Run Simultaneously

Were we born to run?

All signs point to yes.

From his office at Harvard University, Professor of Human Evolutionary Biology Daniel Lieberman says, "Quadrupeds cannot pant and gallop at the same time. Imagine you are chasing a gazelle, a kudu, or some big animal." The so-called "barefoot professor" adds, "If you can chase that animal, make it gallop for 10 to 15 minutes, you've got dinner."*

A friend sent me Dr. Lieberman's video interview on YouTube when I was looking into barefoot running. I have sent the link

---

* Most of the recent examples of followed hunts, called persistence hunting, have recorded animal capture times that took longer than 15 minutes. Some have been recorded at 2 to 6 hours and have taken a group of hunter-trackers.

to most of my fitness and science contacts, who also have been amazed by the barefoot professor's enthralling message. Lieberman says it's not true that you need special shoes to run, "You just need feet."

At present, the rebirth of barefoot running could be categorized as a leading biomechanical discovery of the modern era ... at least my modern era. And this development wasn't produced by going crazy with technology. It was gained by going back in time. All one had to do was watch people who still live something close to hunter-gatherer lifestyles. And see how they run.

Of course, to teach us modernites the engineering and biomechanics of feet and running strides, it's helpful to show us foot impact with slow-mo camera work and voice-overs from credible scientists. Lieberman's Youtube videos provide this.

How Did Humans Decide to Stop Running?

We adults in the West generally stop running at the end of high school. Only about 8 to 10 percent of Americans say they are runners. In one of my core social groups, about three dozen or so people in their 40s to 60s, I know of only two others who say they go jogging on a regular basis. If we stop running, how did we get a healthful, euphoric high? There are a number of ways including dancing, hiking, cycling, spiritual rejoicing, trancelike healing states, family time, yoga, and love making. Don't forget doing nice things for others.

How did the move to sedentary lifestyles arrive on the ancient scene? Did some human tribes run low on wildlife and wild plants? Or, perhaps they decided they didn't want to run as much, or travel as many miles on their gathering missions? Was it because we are programmed to conserve energy?

Whatever the case, circa 9,000 B.C., archaic humans began to grow their own crops and raise their own animals for food. Generally speaking, the more they settled into farming, the more their health deteriorated. This is evidenced in fossil remains that show superior bone density among hunter-gatherers who generally ate a more varied diet and fasted more regularly. Anthropology and archeology are fascinating fields of study. Some of the most useful finds come the era of when hunter-gatherers formed sedentary villages—permanent settlements.

A captivating documentary on the formation of sedentary villages is called "How Art Made The World." Cambridge professor Nigel Spivey, who stars in the documentary, says he was given free rein in the history he chose to depict in the film.

This control enabled Dr. Spivey to artfully portray his hypothesis: that building large temples and statues was part of what caused ancient peoples to require food be brought close to the worksite. Large groups of people needed to be fed, housed, and clothed. In this way, in this professor's view, sedentary villages were born and temples were raised.

As always, don't fret the varied viewpoints you may run across. Use such videos as starting points for your intellectual musings, and keep that grain of salt available. Many a good theory has been disproven over time.

As a rule, when I'm looking for a natural solution, I look to the hunter-gatherers and concentrate on the word "natural." The farmers and the industrialists were the workaday boozers, not the hunter-gatherers. The hunter-gatherers were the more naturally living lot, even for the tribes who had mind-altering substances.

Those who were observed and written about had schedules that were commonly balanced between work, family, and play.

Rock Potatoes

What if people won't budge?

Based on what we know of personality traits, it's likely some tribal members would have preferred to sit around on boulders all day, shirking their responsibilities, twiddling their thumbs, and watching the clouds go by as the nearby plants and animals grew and someone else served them for dinner. Were these select few the original rock potatoes? Would they have bided their time waiting around until a broiled bovine (the one that oinks) was cooked up extra crispy?

If they did, would they be super-sized due to lack of any movement besides jaw and bowel? Would they have descendants?

We do know what happened to the animals raised for food and I will attempt to document this with convincing anecdotal evidence. The historical record shows that in the fun-packed year of 1988, descendants of those two-legged and four-legged domesticated animals wound up on hot platters at restaurants like Sizzler.

As you may have heard, this resulted in lines of hunger-stricken people packing themselves into the restaurant. They were called "average consumers." And the voracious appetite doesn't stop with food. Some of these folks are known to run—even stampede—at least once per year when retail and box stores open for business on Black Friday, the big sales day that occurs the Friday after Thanksgiving.

Of course, it's not just Sizzler. The other proverbial usual suspects were, and still are, providing high-calorie, taste-bud-pleasing meals. These modern meals fire our brain chemistry and salivary glands since they are frequently made using the formula of sugar, fat, and salt. And it doesn't matter if it's at a restaurant, a barbecue, or on a camping stove. The sensors of the human brain are fired by what hits the pallet and lands in the gut. When we smell what's cooking, the message is loud and clear. "Ladies and gentlemen, start your engines."

Consider a significant difference between the post mid-20th-century Westerner and prior agricultural and industrial generations: the easy access to affordable meat. Historically, for urban and suburban dwellers, meat was often expensive and not as easy to come by. What's more, prior generations of course seasoned their meat, but using sugar in the meat recipe was much rarer prior to the second half of the 20th century.

Combine the diet of fat, salt, and sugar, and mix in an extremely sedentary lifestyle, and you get supersized, insulin resistant, diabetic modernites. To make matters worse, these people generally eat too often and too quickly. Such a diet spells stomach distress and likely some HAZMAT vapors. These come in the form of a cloud of methane that can clear out a room.

This new breed of late-20th-century sedentary people didn't need to stay in one communal village. But when they left the confines of their residential drywall boxes, they wanted to be carted around to various destinations by cars, trucks, SUVs, and mass transportation, emphasis on the *mass*. At home, they wanted to remain seated, often reclining or lying down. In fact, their couch or desk console became their royal throne and the channel flipper and its cousin, the computer mouse, became their royal decree. King and queen, we are, of our own castles, studio apartments, and dorm rooms ... when the roomies are gone. The castle is of course protected. For some of us, the garage door opener is our own personal "moat control."

Feeling Decadent?

Eventually, anthropologically speaking, wider-belted humans no longer wanted to run after or raise their own quadrupeds. They just wanted to eat them, with some salted, sugary sauce. And wash it all down with 16-ounces of more sugar and taste—soft drinks or fermented plants, aka alcohol. Beverages, of course, hand restaurants their highest profit margins. And if these customers are feeling *decadent or adventurous* (as the wait staff like to entice), perhaps a 7-ounce piece of pie with whipped cream and cherry sauce could satisfy their cravings. Another classic profit product.

Getting hungry yet?

It's no wonder; that's exactly what food scientists and marketers are paid to do. Getting you salivating, and then buying, gets them promoted. Getting you hooked on a feeling and an image for life means holiday bonuses for the corporate staffer and a messed up diet and addiction for us and our kids. Nearly everywhere we turn, the aisles and shelves are stacked against us.

In his article "Food Fight," best-selling author Michael Pollan proposes, "The medical care crisis probably cannot be addressed without addressing the catastrophe of the American diet, and that diet is the direct (even if unintended) result of the way that our agriculture and food industries have been organized."[40]

How and Why Are Our Farms So Appallingly Modern?

An analyst who tracks agriculture for a living sent me this

incendiary note.

"U.S. farmers were just 1.8 percent of the population in 1990, for example, compared to 39 percent in 1900 and 25 percent in 1935. It's been a long and steady bleed on the government's part to get all of us to move off the farm. That is very important for population management, because historically if there was a depression or war, people could always fall back to the farm to sustain themselves. Now that none of us have access to or knowledge of food, we are totally and completely reliant on the government to save us. That was done by design, over the course of several centuries. The irony is they used depression and war to accelerate the demographic shift, which, in the end, puts us under the control of the Elites."

Now, if the above doesn't shake up your comfortable reading posture ...

Unlike their preceding generations, the couch potatoes no longer needed active physical movement to harvest a plateful of food. Sedentary lifestyles allowed them to be disconnected from that notion up to a point. With a flip of the channel, they could watch others do the moving. Sexy and attractive TV dancers and their VIP partners did enough wonderful movement to satisfy millions of viewers who tuned in to watch "Dancing with the Stars."

"Look at these people move, dear," says one spouse potato to the other. "My grandparents could do moves like that ..." Burp, "Do we have any pizza delivery coupons?"

The Short Look Back for Wisdom

Finding wisdom is one way to improve things in your life. Using it and spreading it are also venerable traditions.

Western people sometimes look back a few generations to

determine what the older, sometimes wiser generations were up to. And they should be encouraged to do so. But don't stop there; keep going back.

The argument could be made that over 99 percent of our roots come from an age-old time of hunting and gathering. In good times this was an age of movement, more downtime, snoozing, and recreation. In bad times it was starvation and dying from exposure. Less than 1 percent of our human roots come from the periods which encompass farming and the much later age of modern industrialization. Great Britain's industrialization began around 1760. The general consensus of the historical record is that plant and animal domestication began around 9,000 B.C.

Upright walking history has been dated to a point between 6 and 7 million years ago. Divide the 12,000 years of farming history by 6 million, and you get .0020, or 0.20 percent, which of course is less than 1 percent. If you use the age of Homo sapiens, the number of years spent in sedentary villages remains minimal compared to those spent roaming and foraging. Use 12,000 again and divide it by 200,000 years, and you get .06 or 6 percent.

So ... maybe 6 percent of our Homo sapiens history has been at least partially living in sedentary villages. Again, sedentary villages mean settlements that remain in the same place (either seasonally or for years), raising plants and animals. It's important to remind that hunting and gathering continued in most farming societies. Where I grew up in still rural New Jersey, we hunted deer and pheasants right in and along the acres of corn stalks and fields of winter rye grass. Today, people still do. These days, as has been explained to me, the cornfields in my home county in rural New Jersey are mostly planted with GMO corn. That generally means the corn is resistant to herbicides that are now part of the soil composition and water runoff—egads.

The point here is that ancient and modern Homo sapiens in the West moved their masses even though they lived in sedentary villages. These movers continued to move up until the mid-20th century. They also ate less processed and chemically laced food. Then everything changed.

Now consider the Industrial Age. In years, less than 1 percent of Homo sapiens history was part of this era. In historical terms, sedentism and the Industrial Age are so innovatively recent, they stand as new things for human beings and the planet to contend with.

Skulls and Bones of Old

There are ranges of explanations and beliefs about the origins of our species. Consider two of the oldest identified fossils. Toumaï is a skull discovered in 2001 in Chad that has both apelike and humanlike features. This find, dating between 6 and 7 million years ago, is currently the oldest known fossil considered to be of the family hominine. This group is made up of humans, gorillas, chimpanzees, and bonobos.

Ardi, a 45-percent-complete skeleton discovered in Ethiopia in 1994, dates back 4.4 million years and shows that her species walked upright but had a grasping big toe for climbing trees.

With just a peek into ancient anthropology, we can take away an important perception. The farming and industrial communities of our recent past are such miniscule portions of hominid history.*

Oz's Cowardly Lion sings, "What do they got that I ain't got?"

If a resident of the new millennium were to ask this of a scholar on hunter-gatherers, the answer might be downtime.

Downtime is time spent doing things like arts and crafts, bonding with peers, watching kids play, resting, reading, and recreating. Already mentioned were walking and jogging if they are releases for you. If you want to know about your distant ancestors' history of survival, healthful living, and afternoons of downtime, look back to the life of hunter-gatherers. It wasn't Woodstock or one of today's Earth-friendly intentional communities. But when there was food and water, when they were free of invading marauders, when the elements weren't wreaking unbearable wrath, this group of humans certainly seemed to have spent a fair amount of time living what could be called happy and harmonious lives. We just don't know if the extinct members were able to carry a tune or hit a high C during a primal scream.

As previously mentioned, history had its share of malaise. The Native Americans had their scalpers and torturers like Red Cloud and his band. There were times marked by a certain impermanency of peace and harmony for hunter-gatherers. If you have ever spent time out in the elements, you'll understand the obvious threats. There were likely always times in one's life of near-constant worry about food, shelter, weather, and defense.

---

* Hominids are upright-walking primates whose family includes Homo sapiens and Homo erectus as well as other extinct species, so categorized for their increased brain size, intelligence, and smaller jaws and teeth. They are considered the direct predecessors of modern humans.

Romancing the Stone

Living in the wild has a certain romantic ring to it. The bodies of hunter-gatherers shown in photography and film depict people who look quite capable. Many of those caught on film are also shown frequently smiling.

Compare that to paunchy commuters listening to news radio stuck in rush-hour traffic on the New Jersey Turnpike, sipping on a pint of designer coffee to wash down antacid pills. Picture this and you may appreciate how the Paleo Movement took the West by storm.

Authors and journalists are capturing strategies of a sub-cultural swing toward what some consider healthful pursuits of the Pleistocene and Paleolithic periods that lasted from roughly 2.5 million years ago to some 11,700 years ago—the advent of agriculture. The Paleo converts claim our bodies are maladapted to handle high consumption of carbs and the highly processed foods. Instead, thinking back to the Stone-Age people, some believers in Paleo look to a diet that has some or a lot of natural meat including the bones and connective tissue. Bones can be stewed to extract collagen-building materials from tendons, the stem cells from the marrow, and important amino acids like proline and glycine. Add some vegetables and seasonings to the stew *et voila*. Stew is about by far the most complete, easy, cooked meal to prepare. And, for many of us, it's easier than digging up grubs. I have yet to meet a Paleo convert who claims to eat grubs and worms but I'm sure some do.

Numbers of the Paleo folks also suggest getting plenty of exercise (especially high intensity training), outdoor time, barefoot time, and purification from nature. Some even hold to owning fewer personal belongings. Look up the Simplicity Movement for more on that.

Paleofantasy?

Marlene Zuk writes about this back-to-old-school or stone-school movement in her book "Paleofantasy." Her book makes a good case for the argument that it's impossible to go back. Tell that to the luxury-bred Roman elite, some of whom had to survive in the wild after Rome fell during a prolonged attack of starvation. Seeing hungry, surviving Romans in the fields and woods meant it was likely no grub was safe for hundreds of miles. No farmers' fields or women were either ... if a former senator-turned-highway-bandit happened to turn up. "Mad Max"-type stories have occurred a multitude of times in history and those stories are mentioned in religious texts.

No matter what the historical record shows, it seems obvious that the lifestyles of some prior generations tend to get sentimental-ized. Our innate cultural curiosity begs the question: Who indeed lived better lives? Are we modernites taking psychotropic drugs simply because we have them available? Would large numbers of hunter-gatherers have been hooked on such substances? Is it accurate to put forward that any survivalist commune would have perished if they got hooked on a substance or practice that compromised their ability to survive? What was in those peace pipes anyway?

Try to shoot an arrow or set a snare while brain impaired and see how you do. Online videos show a bizarre activity called drunk boxing, where participants down quantities of alcohol before fighting each other. In such contests, the participants spend much of their time falling down and getting up and then throwing big punches that miss, causing them to again fall down.

When it comes to anthropological lifestyle comparisons, one erudite person to consider is UCLA professor Jared Diamond who has done extensive work in this field. He has spent decades chronicling and verbally sharing his findings on the lives of the ancients. He and others paint a picture of communal cooperation enjoyed by the hunter-gatherers who generally rose at dawn and bedded down at sunset.

These people weren't wired to the electric matrix like we are, and they weren't clicking away at their thumb boards and keyboards with their heads down and their postures slouched. Their physicality was part of their survival and euphoria. I for one think life would be dull without some regular, if not daily, euphoric moments. Then there's the ethic of freedom which finds more footing with the barefoot and moccasin-shod than it does with the pack rats of the industrial world—so many of whom live one paycheck or government check away from eviction.

This isn't to suggest that evolution hasn't *naturally* put us exactly where we are. The human drive to make life easier and safer has indeed placed the residents of the industrial world inside drywall with microwave cooking. I do take issue with Dr. Zuk's point of view about the over-rated downtime of hunter-gatherers. Some assuredly had it more abundantly than we—starting with the Hawaiians in certain epochs.

Many researchers and writers have lived with specific groups of the modern hunter-gatherers who had ample food supplies and lived close to fresh water. Some have relayed positive stories that demonstrate how some tribes handle work and chores in far fewer hours than many of us do. The acceptable assertion from my reading is that as a group, we generally have less individual and communal downtime than the ancients—again, given access to food, water, and a cooperating climate. A crystal ball of tribal lore would reveal that more stuff equates to more chores. Non-farming tribal people are minimalists and minimalism provides its own type of convenience.

For the established modernite, how easy is it to locate a needed item among the boxes in the garage or basement? How convenient is it for you to take your computer or phone in for servicing? Just managing all of our stuff takes an exorbitant amount of time. If you look at your schedule for the month you may see how plenty of your supposed non-work hours were taken up by something quite the opposite of free time or downtime.

Today, people are communing—not necessarily to live together but definitely to build community and end the disconnection we have from one another. There's carpooling, ridesharing, bike sharing, communal meals, CouchSurfing, Meetup.com, and even house swapping. They are setting up more and more opportunities for group gatherings—even if some take place online. Then there's the call of nature. Some of us have access to nature, while many others must admit to a shortfall of time spent in the great outdoors. For most of us in the West, "time away" from the grind takes lots of time and money.

To hit a bit harder, one observation has it that we sit on our rumps inside boxes of mass media and corporate culture, stuck in the presence of others addicted to sedentism, living far less communally than many prior generations. The nomadic tribes, whose goal was to set up camps with shelter before nightfall, might look at our lives in this way: *Industrial societies of today flock to an overabundance of shelter and collectibles.* Compared to them, we're all hoarders. How much time do you spend indoors? How many belongings do you have in boxes you rarely open or storage facilities you dread visiting.

The wellness movement is fighting some of this evolution and these excessive human tendencies. If the laws of attraction are applicable, the digital screen seems the most potent magnet since the loincloth.

Life is a series of karmic reprisals and rewards. Some things, as well as people, draw us in—possibly due to these same laws of attraction. Then there's past life regression, the unconscious mind, and good old performance anxiety. We have to deal with lots of things these days—even loneliness. More people are living alone than ever before. Are you alone, or lonely? Of course these two words are not the same.

Some of us may not believe it takes a village to raise a child. Examples show a vigilant and lucky single parent can do it. But wouldn't it be a lot more rewarding to take care of the village and assist each other in a communal way? Wouldn't it be nice to get a breather from your day instead of being inundated with heavy responsibility and go-go-go? I grew up with extended family assisting in childcare, meal preparation, and the sharing of wisdom. Raising kids on our own is a balancing act whose risk is frequently placed on one or two key people. Do you really believe this recently fashionable custom is the right way to proceed?

When it comes to spinning media stories and funding advertising campaigns, do you think it makes sense to continue to trip people up with half truths, false imagery, and sabotage? If not, is the dog-eat-dog world ready for a remedy of rational thought, natural healing, and cooperation?

Easy Takeaways

1. "The media never met a new study it didn't like."

2. Bedtime hour and melatonin levels are principal determinants for wakeup hour.

3. The tribe people of the Tarahumara in the outback Copper Canyon of Mexico run with joy, not with grimacing faces of exhaustion.

4. "Growing your own food is a dangerous act because you're in danger of becoming free."

5. The homininae were movers and we can learn much from watching how they lived, especially the bonobos who are the most peaceful and individually long-lived of any of the Great Apes.

6. Could "Mad Max" survivalist lifestyles become part of the West's 21st century?

Chapter 8

The Sifu Slim Program for Daily Living

Be coachable and seek out good coaches.

Take a moment to list five of the best coaches, teachers, and mentors you've had. Include what they helped you with. If you are in need of one, feel free to join me for an upcoming webinar. You know, online coaching. Believe me, it works; I tap into good coaches myself.

1. _____

2. _____

3. _____

4. _____

5. _____

"No matter what accomplishments you make,
somebody helped you."
—Althea Gibson, the first African-American tennis player
(a woman) to win a Grand Slam event—1956 French Open.
(1927 Clarendon County, S.C. – 2003 East Orange, N.J.)

The Way

Ob as cha miad, is Farsi for *water comes from the well.* This is a direct statement that makes sense to most. Likewise, good health comes from doing healthful things. *Euphoros,* is the Greek word for health which leads to joy and elation. These are the essential parts of a healthful program for a healthful lifestyle.

There are ways to grow an organic garden by keeping the soil and worms happy and well fed. What is a good way to grow your body and mind? Tap into the superior health of tribal peoples and their propensity for having downtime. Don't work at jobs that endlessly culminate in fifteen-hour days, even if they are your passion. At least avoid making days go that long on a regular basis. If you must work long days, mix in the parts of this program you can stick to. In the promotion of balance it's important to remind that kicks and retrogrades cause extreme vacillation in looks and health—not to mention moodiness. The following are some aspects of my daily lifestyle of wellness. This draws upon millennia of wisdom and a realistic look at the sedentary state of today's daily life.

The Sifu Slim Program for Daily Living

(This is what I have found works for my schedule and need for functionality. See what works for your needs. I will say this, if I do daily physical activity, I have a good chance at handling stress and making it through the tougher days. As we all know, the worried mind trapped inside a sedentary body can wreak all kinds of havoc, no matter what kind of day we face.)

1. Fitness and mind connection every morning, normally outdoors. I do one to two hours depending on schedule and energy level. Thirty minutes is my absolute minimum, and I usually only do a program that short if I have something else physical scheduled for later. Type A's, watch your propensity for stacking a litany of things to complete that have to be done "no matter what."

2. Vary things by day. On one day, I may do a program of warm-ups and functional training followed by barefoot sprints up a grass incline. I may then do coordinated crawling (in all four directions—forward, backward, sideways left and right) on flat terrain. The sprints are focused and smooth. The crawling (sometimes called "bear crawls" or "monkey crawls" because it's not on the knees) is not about speed but about maintaining good form. I like to do these wearing my grippy gloves that are sometimes called "moving or gardening gloves." For a fit and agile person, the crawling can be done on any surface—asphalt, grass, sand. The idea is to be smooth and agile, not rough.

3. On other days, I start out with functional training (structural support strengthening similar to Pilates); and then biomechanical exercises (alignment and strengthening exercises that were personally prescribed for my personal posture by a biomechanical practitioner); then yoga poses; and stretches. Then it's on to bar exercises like chin-ups and bodyweight shoulder presses; and what I call martial-artsy

calisthenics: a mix of a martial arts warm up and high school P.E. calisthenics. I do most all this in a Zen-like state. It would seemingly get too boring doing this for decades without heightened spirits. I hit most every area from head to toe and even do neck and facial exercises.

4. The face, abs, hips, grip, and dynamic stretching (including unweighted good-mornings) I normally do every day.

5. At least one day per week, I do an extended endurance program plus some of the aforementioned exercises. Detailing this, I do one long run, hike, bike, or recreational event, often on the weekend. My long run or bike ride plus the accompanying outdoor workout normally goes for two to three hours. The aerobic portion of this goes between 40 minutes and three hours. Three hours of aerobics means I'm probably hiking. In my life, I have run, with short periodic stops for a drink, for two hours at a clip. At times my body's connective tissue is not happy if I run for more than 40 minutes or so. Sometimes it does just fine. Our body is moody, that's just the way it is.

6. I don't expect most readers to have this level of fitness/commitment to wellness, but if you want to see the *correct* technique for these exercises and to determine which of them is the best fit *for your lifestyle,* you can download or order videos at *MaintenanceWorkout.com.*

7. To the four directions of the compass, I bow-out at the end of every workout, honoring the space and what I have given and received. I also give a blessing (prayer, giving thanks, acknowledging family, those in need, and planet, higher power, etc.) at each meal.

---

8. I eat mostly high-quality, tasty food. To me, even quality broccoli is tasty. I have a voracious appetite, but I do fast at times for reasons of health, energy, digestive repair, and focus. It's good to be able to metabolize your fat stores which we all have. Your body knows how to tap into its own fat stores. Can you stop eating long enough to allow your body to do this? Contrary to what I learned previously, I now frequently don't eat immediately after exercise or physical exertion. I normally exercise from 5 to 7 a.m. and frequently don't eat an official meal until a few hours later. This has provided me more energy, clearer mind, toxic cleansing, less gutty look, and better digestive processing.

9. Drink water all day long. I cycle in squeezed fruits which are low in sugar—grapefruit and lemons are exceptionally low in sugar. Cutting in all the pulp is great for taste and health. These two citrus fruits neutralize excess intestinal (and thus systemic) acidity. Eat some of the rind; it's wonderfully rich in fiber and nutrients. For storing liquids, glass bottles are best. Lately I have been using the containers Knudsen's organic juices come in. At times I add cinnamon, known for these properties: taste, antibacterial, anti-inflammatory, blood pressure regulating, blood-sugar level regulating, aphrodisiacal. Caveat with cinnamon: Some experts say it should be used in small quantities (less than half a teaspoon). Test it and see. Refrain from taking it if it causes you any side effects like stomach distress. Refrain from taking it if you are on other medication. Tea was once another favorite thirst quencher. For those who are predisposed to problems with alcohol consumption,

note there is a link between caffeine consumption and cravings for alcohol. Fortunately, I've never craved alcohol. A few years ago, I decreased my tea consumption drastically and have found this of benefit to general health. At times I do drop a whole stalk of mint and basil directly into my water bottle. Presto—garden fresh herbal tea. Keep up your guard with food products produced and shipped in bulk. Productions done on large scales are generally compromised in some respects. The specifics on this would fill a book.

10. Work at a fulfilling job. If you can't find one, have faith. Revel in the difficulty of completing tasks you don't necessarily enjoy doing. Accomplishment typically means doing hard tasks. This can propel you to rejoice in a task's completion as well as enhance your free time. Take baby steps.

11. Naps and downtime as needed and when possible. I generally take five to seven naps per week. Hallelujah! My parents mandated we three kids take naps when we were little. How else were they going to have their romantic time and bonus rest?

12. Stretch period before sleeping. If I'm tired, I'll do it before dinner. Then I'll eat dinner and then be a couch relaxer, not a potato.

13. I'm in bed between 8:30 and 9:30 p.m. during the weekdays. I read a bit, then sleep until between 4 and 5:30 a.m. Around seven hours of sleep for me at night plus between 30 minutes and one hour allotted for a weekday siesta. You will know how many hours of sleep are right for your rhythms. If you don't, chart it out yourself, or go

see a sleep specialist. Weekends are great for long, midday or afternoon snoozes. Once in a while, based on my body's needs, I'll drift off to bed early and get in an extra hour or two of sleep.

14. Affection and lovemaking on a regular basis. This is part of emotional health and a significant part of the glue that holds a couple's relationship together. The expression of love is something I'd chose not to live without. Deep, committed love can endure and make life wonderful.

Once You're There, You're There

Physical mastery is not drudgery; it's a joy. Once you are fit, well, and happy, the healthy lifestyle becomes so easy and rewarding that you can't live without it. It's euphoric and enthralling. But remember, if you have been unfit for a while, you probably won't arrive at the pleasure zone, the optimum level, for a while—in some cases, quite a while. When you get there, you will have to grow accustomed to being there. Patience is a virtue. It's not about the destination; it's about the journey.

To avoid self-sabotage, accept the new you in the new surroundings you have created. Until you can truly accept this with open arms, until you love that new place, you are vulnerable to missing out on the experience. You are also at risk of falling off the smooth-riding wagon.

Think of the final moment this way. When you have made it, you are the smooth wet sand at low tide—clean, optimally formed, and available to others who may want to jog through or stand on the stable ground to look to fish or simply look out. You're ready for action and whatever life throws at you.

But remember, the tides come back daily—about two times in fact—and may deposit all kinds of debris. Think of this natural refuse and washed up human garbage as the stress.

If your beach is clean and prepared for the incoming tide and ready to handle the new load of demands and stresses, the sandy path will deposit manageable levels of new debris. That natural debris may again be taken out with the falling tide and provide organic matter for the sea's creatures.

If your beach is overly inundated with yesterday's debris, now you've got two loads of debris to deal with. A week of this and you have a clogged up, smelly beach. Now the beach needs transformation. It's off maintenance. Two months of this repetitive stress and now it needs a major overhaul. Ten years of living like this as a middle-aged human might mean a post-op week in a hospital and a lengthy recovery. If you practice maintenance, you *will* see and feel results. If you backslide, don't give up. Take it day by day, setting a daily goal until health becomes habit. My daily fitness goal is simple: Do an outdoor morning routine that invigorates the mind, body, and spirit. And take short stretch breaks on the hour, mixing in some jumping jacks or rope skipping when appropriate. Keep your lymph moving. Don't let the human cesspool stagnate.

Get With It

When a person changes their deeply entrenched values about health and wellness, amazing things start to happen. When you accept a new philosophy of euphoria you become a new person—healthful to the core. When you master it, you become a master.

Like most of us in the "free" world, you were probably subjected to a Westernized attempt to program you—to make you a *cookie-cutter rules follower*. It seems that so few these days got their programming to be seekers and outright discoverers. I'm here to tell you it won't be until you create the time, and instill in yourself the will to go on a quest for this discovery, that you will find the true meaning of the maintenance and wellness philosophy being offered.

Reading this book is an invitation for you to start a journey. While on that journey, you will have the opportunity to gain a greater realization of what true wellness and happiness are. You will also get to know yourself—the new, more relaxed and enlightened, invigorated, and accepting you. You might even become more huggable and lovable.

> *"Now and then it's good to pause*
> *in our pursuit of happiness and just be happy."*
> —Guillaume Apollinaire (1880 Rome – 1910 Paris)

Just don't equate fast food or junk food with happiness. That is what some of these corporations' major shareholders have been watching people do. As they reel in dividends that your spending habits provide, some of these shareholders may consider you not only a patron but also a guinea pig for their latest unhealthful product line.

What Is Your Philosophy If You Can't Articulate It?

By that I mean, what is your philosophy if you can't write it down or speak it in a plain manner?

The answer to me is obvious: few words and lots of doing. Since actions speak louder than words, the message is delivered through your actions.

You can simply live it, live out your philosophy. Show by doing;

teach by doing. Once you have the base, you will know you have it, and you will know it works. You'll know because others will witness it and perhaps even be intrigued.

What this book offers over all else in the way of actionable steps is *how to* acquire a new viewpoint based on age-old wisdom and your life's experiences. I promise you that this philosophy, together with its evolving and adapting temperament, works ... because I live it. And so have a long list of fitness pioneers, including Jack LaLanne, Bonnie Prudden, and B.K.S Iyengar—a yoga master from India who passed away at age 95. Both Jack and Bonnie made it into their late 90s with lots of health, prosperity, humor, and good times. I'm also a follower of another man known for his silly side. Bruce Lee, an icon of fitness, martial arts, film, and the modern era raised the bar for what it means to push human potential.

He passed away at age 32 partially because of being more performance oriented than wellness minded. He suffered a broken back while doing squats which led to an addiction to painkillers and an eventual early demise. One could make the case that his life was long out of balance. That he was winding down as he was winding up. One could also make the case that he did what he did exceptionally well and had completed more in 32 years than many of us will do in 95. Those interested in reading about lifestyles of balance can review my work at The Aging Athlete Project.

This system of beliefs combines wisdom from over 6 million years of hunter-gatherer existence with new operating directions to follow in the modern sedentary nations.

You may not know if it works until you perfect it. Then, and only then, may you embrace the true gift of the program. But for you newbies who want some form of initial results, rest assured, you should feel a little better after your first day of practice.

The Intentions

In writing Sedentary Nation, the intention was to make it readable, interesting, understandable, autobiographical, educational, and motivational. In short, a book that works for you when you work with it. The effort was to take a look at wellness in the new millennium—where there has been an attempt to compartmentalize its pieces—and provide what may be a more holistic approach to wellness in a computer-centric, *busy* world. You, the reader, will be the judge of whether I've succeeded or not.

The participants whom I have found do the best with wellness are those who make their own personal commitment and then adhere to that commitment for the rest of their lives. And they do it with these added bonuses: They embrace the wonderful pastime of physical recreation, and they get high on their own natural euphoria.

As for citations on that, simply quote Sifu Slim, Sedentary Nation.

I encourage you to welcome openness and wellness into your lives. If I can help in any way, please let me know. Through the media, public speaking, workshops, and Internet webinars, I welcome the opportunity to bring my wellness message to your particular group. Until we again connect, remember,

"Life is like riding a bicycle—
in order to keep your balance, you must keep moving."
—Albert Einstein (1879 Ulm, Kingdom of Württemberg,
German Empire – 1955 Princeton, New Jersey)

Here's to our happy days, together ...

Honor life, honor it all.
Sifu Slim, Santa Bárbara, California

Easy Takeaways

1. Be coachable and seek out good coaches.

2. Vary your exercise program for a comprehensive approach that maintains your total body and brain health as well as your interest.

3. Patience is a virtue.

4. "Now and then it's good to pause in our pursuit of happiness and just be happy."

5. Demonstrate your health philosophy with few words and lots of doing. Actions speak louder than words.

6. Embrace the wonderful pastime of physical recreation and learn to get high on your own natural euphoria.

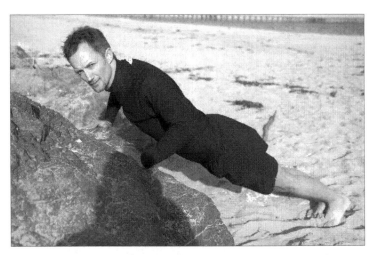

The author's creed—no gym is needed for the hunter-gatherer, martial arts outdoor workout.

About the Author

Sifu Slim is a Jack LaLanne mixed with Bruce Lee trapped inside the body of Gilligan. Sifu Slim (Henry Kreuter) is an author, wellness educator/speaker,lifelong amateur athlete, and leading proponent of "intentionalphysical activity." Sifu (pron. See Foo) is Cantonese for father-teacher or master. Sifu has developed easy-to-follow programs to empower everyone to achieve more healthful lifestyles and an instinctive wellness mindset. Inspired by legendary fitness icon Jack LaLanne, Sifu has made it his life's mission to promote "maintenance fitness," which makes physical activity both recreational and joyful, and a routine part of our daily lives.

Consider Sifu as a resource for your group's wellness needs—in English, French, or Spanish. He is roadshow ready, webinar literate, and media ops fluent. Sifu is also the author of "The Aging Athlete," see *TheAgingAthlete.com*, a crash course on the persistence of the human spirit. By gaining the trust of an impressive cross-section of today's modern athletes and seasoned veterans, Sifu Slim provides readers with an insider's look at the heart and mind—and even the soul—of top performers from football, basketball, body building, triathlon, swimming, track, martial arts, MMA fighting, and distance running.

The research for this book revealed that the unique individuals who dedicate their lives to honing their bodies in the pursuit of excellence share an undeniable kinship with us all. Their captivating personal experiences and hard won triumphs in overcoming life's obstacles will resonate with anyone interested in living a fully realized, purposeful existence. The athletes featured inspire us to live the realizable dream of perpetual health and fitness.

Do you know any interesting aging male and female
former top athletes who are still maintaining their fitness
and who would be interested in sharing their story
for a future book?

Contact: TheAgingAthlete.com

"The Aging Athlete will help you unlock potential
in your mind that can significantly impact your overall well-being.
Its insights, logic, and practicality are outstanding. This book is
meaningful, timeless, and profound."
—Dr. Jarrod Spencer, Sports Psychologist,
Mind of the Athlete, LLC

Coupons

As discounts are available these offers may apply:
- Go to MaintenanceWorkout.com
- Click on DVDs
- Select a DVD
- Click on the order form.
- Type this into the CODE BOX:

havingagreatdayofmovement

And you may be eligible for a percentage off your purchase of a fitness DVD.

To buy a discounted copy Sedentary Nation:
- Go to SedentaryNation.com
- Type this into the CODE BOX:

upandoffthecouch

And you may be eligible for a percentage off.

To buy a discounted copy of The Aging Athlete:
- Go To TheAgingAthlete.com
- Find the personal, proprietary website.
- Click on the order form.
- Type this into the CODE BOX:
- Whoisstillfitthesedays

All discounts are subject to change

and dependent on availability.

TheAgingAthlete.com

SedentaryNation.com

Endnotes

1   Websters online <http://www.merriam-webster.com/dictionary/prostrate>
2   Gabe Johnson and Emily Weinstein, "Navigating the Aisles." New York Times documentary video on Youtube. April 30 2013. <https://www.youtube.com/watch?v=ATAZrRfebiw>
3   From excerpted portion of Chapter 1 of "120 Years of American Education: A Statistical Portrait" (Edited by Tom Snyder, National Center for Education Statistics, 1993). <http://nces.ed.gov/naal/lit_history.asp>
4   <http://www.cdc.gov/nchs/data/lifetables/life1890-1910.pdf>
5   Roni Caryn Rabin, "Risks: Side Effects Fueled by High-Energy Drinks." New York Times. February 2011 <http://www.nytimes.com/2011/02/15/health/research/15risks.html>
6   Herizo Evo, "5 Habits That Are Good To Do Before Sleep." Articles of Health Care Inc., July 7, 2013. <http://www.articlesofhealthcare.com/971/5-habits-that-are-good-to-do-before-sleep/>
7   Sarah Novak, "Rise and Shine: New Study Finds Morning Larks Are Consistently Happier Than Night Owls." Discovery Fit & Health, June 12, 2012. <http://blogs.discovery.com/dfh-sara-novak/2012/06/rise-and-shine-new-study-finds-morning-larks-are-consistently-happier-than-night-owls.html>
8   Professor Mark J. Perry's Blog for Economics and Finance, May 2, 2010. <http://mjperry.blogspot.com/2010/05/more-tv-sets-than-people-per-household.html>
9   Dan Buettner, "The Secrets of Long Life." National Geographic, 2005. <http://ngm.nationalgeographic.com/print/2005/11/longevity-secrets/buettner-text> as well as other sources.

10 Selene Yeager, "Sitting is the New Smoking – Even for Runners." Runner's World, July 20, 2013. <http://www.runnersworld.com/health/sitting-is-the-new-smoking-even-for-runners?page=single>

11 Ron Winslow, "The Guide to Beating a Heart Attack." WSJ.com. April 16, 2012 <http://online.wsj.com/article/SB10001424052702304818404577347982400815676.html>

12 SBCC Adult Education Seminar by Dr. David Beamer.

13 Julie Newberg, ASU ergonomics site addresses proper workplace practices. ASU News, June 5, 2012. <https://asunews.asu.edu/20120605_ergonomics percent2520>

14 Corey Washington, "Study Shows Black Children Consuming More Media; Mobile Tech Contributes." June 8, 2011. <http://www.blackvoicenews.com/bvn-now/the-tech-report/46287-study-shows-black-children-consuming-more-media-mobile-technology-contributes.html>

15 Mike Esterl, "Coke Tailors Its Soda Sizes Backing Off of 'Supersizing,' Company Aims for Wider Range of Ounces, Prices." WSJ.com. September 19, 2011. <http://online.wsj.com/article/SB10001424053111903374004576578980270401662.html>

16 Plenty of helpful research and history of the Tour de France is available on the Web and in print. Of particular help to me was a book called "The Tour de France: A Cultural History" by Christopher S. Thompson. University of California Press, 2008.

17 Ann Louise Gittleman and her quote of telecommunications pioneer Clint Ober as included in Gittleman's book "Zapped." Harper One, 2010. p. 71.

18 Camille Sweeney, "Seeking Self-Esteem Through Surgery." NY Times, January 14, 2009. <http://www.nytimes.com/2009/01/15/fashion/15skin.html?_r=0>

19 Frank M. Sacks, M.D., George A. Bray, M.D., et al. "Comparison of Weight-Loss Diets with Different Compositions of Fat, Protein, and Carbohydrates." N Engl J Med 2009; 360:859-873 <http://www.nejm.org/doi/full/10.1056/NEJMoa0804748#t=articleResults>

20 Dave Mason, "It's in our nature-Author says it's good for our minds, bodies and souls to get outside." Santa Barbara News Press. p. D8. May 2, 2012. The first three points are excerpted from Dave Mason's article as above. Points four and five are excerpted from Richard Louv's book, "The

Nature Principle: Reconnecting with Live in a Virtual Age." Algonquin Books, 2011.

21 In 2004, the U.S. EPA banned CCA, Chromated copper arsenate, for use as a pesticide compound in residential use, see <http://www.pollutionissues.com/A-Bo/Arsenic.html>

22 Dan Buettner, Blue Zones. Washington D.C., The National Geographic Society, 2012. p. 62.

23 Andrew T. Ludlow and Stephen M. Roth. "Physical Activity and Telomere Biology: Exploring the Link." with Aging-Related Disease Prevention. Journal of Aging Research. Volume 2011. <http://www.hindawi.com/journals/jar/2011/790378/>

24 Ann Lukits, "Years of Sitting on the Job Linked to Cancer." June 21, 2011. The Wall Street Journal. p. D4,

25 <http://www.merriam-webster.com/dictionary/rest?show=0&t=1372639693>

26 Morbidity and Mortality Weekly Report, Centers for Disease Control and Prevention. December 03, 1999 / 48(47);1073-1080 <http://www.cdc.gov/mmwr/preview/mmwrhtml/mm4847a1.htm>

27 News Release from UCSB Office of Public Affairs. "Hunter-Gatherers, Forager-Horticulturalists Demonstrate Minimal Hypertension and Lower Risk of Heart Disease." May 21, 2012. Study by Michael Gurven et. al. <http://www.ia.ucsb.edu/pa/display.aspx?pkey=2727> Viewed December 2012

28 Raymond Obomsawin, "Historical and Scientific Perspectives on the Health of Canada's First Peoples." March, 2007. p 39 <http://www.soilandhealth.org/02/0203cat/020335.obomsawin.pdf>

29 Harvard University publishes The Harvard Mental Health Letter and included a terrific article on addiction in their July 2004 edition. <http://www.health.harvard.edu/newsweek/The_addicted_brain.htm>

30 This is an excerpt of an article on the Bragg website. The article references this as the source. Jack LaLanne, still strong at 91, attacks child obesity. Associated Press. October 29, 2005. <http://bragg.com/about/lalanne_gospel.html> Viewed April 2013

31 Michael d'Estries, "Jack LaLanne: The first fitness superhero." The Mother Nature Network. January 24th, 2011. <http://www.mnn.com/health/fitness-wellbeing/blogs/jack-lalanne-the-first-fitness-superhero>

32 <http://www.utne.com/Environment/Fast-Food-Culinary-Ethos.aspx#ixzz1Dh4A5DvL>

33 Isaac Osborne, Egoscue Therapist, Santa Barbara, CA. email response. January 27, 2011.

34 See <http://fitlife.tv/1-man-produced-6000-pounds-of-food-on-110-acre/>

35 Daniel Lieberman, "The Story of the Human Body." New York: Pantheon Books, 2013. p. 136.

36 Frans de Waal, "Our Inner Ape." New York: Riverhead Books, 2005 CD 4

37 See The Journal Proceedings of the Royal Society B: Biological Sciences, 2006. <http://rspb.royalsocietypublishing.org/content/273/1598/2177.full.pdf> and also this article by C. Clairborne Ray in the NY Times <http://www.nytimes.com/2012/05/22/science/why-are-chimps-stronger-than-humans.html?_r=0>

38 Richard Ingham, "Did Neanderthals and modern humans co-exist?" IOL Scitech. September 2005. <http://www.iol.co.za/scitech/technology/did-neanderthals-and-modern-humans-co-exist-1.252307>

39 Interview of Daniel Lieberman by Nature Video Channel. 2009. <http://www.youtube.com/watch?v=7jrnj-7YKZE>

40 Michael Pollan, The New York Review of Books, Sept - Oct 2010, no 161.

The Athletes Recovery Getaway

Sifu Slim and a number of his contacts in the health and wellness field have established The Athletes Recovery Getaway, aka TARGwell. Run as a cooperative of many different professionals, the group works with athletes of all ages who seek to get help in a variety of ways.

Sifu is the point person for the athletes who can call and schedule dates for their stays in Santa Barbara, home to world class training centers, medical facilities, and healing opportunities. The intentions: Prevention, Intervention, Rehabilitation, Performance Improvement, Coaching, Goal Setting, Skills Learning, and Rejoicing.

For more information, please email TARGwell@gmail.com

52760260R00192

Made in the USA
San Bernardino, CA
29 August 2017